Bladder Pain Syndrome – An Evolution

Philip M. Hanno • Jørgen Nordling
David R. Staskin • Alan J. Wein
Jean Jacques Wyndaele
Editors

Bladder Pain Syndrome – An Evolution

Springer

Editors
Philip M. Hanno
Stanford University School of Medicine
Stanford, CA
USA

Jørgen Nordling
Department of Urology
Herlev Hospital
Herlev
Denmark

David R. Staskin
St. Elizabeth's Medical Center
Tufts University School of Medicine
Boston, MA
USA

Alan J. Wein
Penn Medicine
Perelman School of Medicine
Perelman Center for Advanced Medicine
University of Pennsylvania Health System
Philadelphia, PA
USA

Jean Jacques Wyndaele
Urology
Antwerp University, GGW
Wilrijk, Antwerp
Belgium

This Book is a second edition to the book 'Interstitial Cystitis' published in 1990
ISBN 978-3-319-87082-3 ISBN 978-3-319-61449-6 (eBook)
https://doi.org/10.1007/978-3-319-61449-6

Printed on acid-free paper

This Springer imprint is published by Springer Nature
The registered company is Springer International Publishing AG
The registered company address is: Gewerbestrasse 11, 6330 Cham, Switzerland

Contents

1 Introduction 1
Philip Hanno, David Staskin, Alan Wein, Jørgen Nordling, and Jean Jacques Wyndaele

2 Historical Perspectives 3
Jane Meijlink

3 The Epidemiology of Interstitial Cystitis/Bladder Pain Syndrome (IC/BPS): How Good Was a Study of 30-Years Ago 11
Philip J. Held, Philip Hanno, and Frank McCormick

4 Epidemiology Commentary 23
J. Curtis Nickel

5 The Prevalence of Bladder Pain Syndrome/Interstitial Cystitis in Italy: The importance of a National Registry 27
Loredana Nasta

6 Interstitial Cystitis: Animal Models 33
Tony Buffington, Michael R. Ruggieri, and David J. Klumpp

7 Etiology: Etiological and Pathogenic Theories of Interstitial Cystitis/Bladder Pain Syndrome 37
Jørgen Nordling, David Staskin, and Naoki Yoshimura

8 Differences in Clinical Features and Histopathology in BPS/IC with and without Hunner Lesions 41
Christina Kåbjörn-Gustafsson and Ralph Peeker

9 Mast Cells and Interstitial Cystitis 49
Frank Aldenborg, Magnus Fall, and Lennart Enerbäck

10 Mast Cells as Biomarkers for Bladder Pain Syndrome/Interstitial Cystitis? 51
Marianne Gamper, Sigrid Regauer, and Volker Viereck

11 Diagnosis of Interstitial Cystitis: A Clinical, Endoscopic and Pathologic Approach 57
Joop P. van de Merwe

12 **Diagnosis of Interstitial Cystitis: A Comment on Glomerulations** 63
Gjertrud Egge Wennevik

13 **Diagnosis of Interstitial Cystitis** 65
Jörgen Quaghebeur

14 **Commentary on Sant Chapter: 30 Years on!** 69
Grannum R. Sant

15 **Neuro-Urologic Evaluation in Interstitial Cystitis** 73
Jean Jacques Wyndaele

16 **Current Role of Neurourologic Evaluation in Interstitial Cystitis/Bladder Pain Syndrome** 77
Hann-Chorng Kuo

17 **Neurourological Evaluation in BPS** 81
Arndt van Ophoven

18 **Bladder Hydrodistension in 2017** 83
Claus Riedl

19 **Pharmacologic Goals in Interstitial Cystitis/Bladder Pain Syndrome** 87
Antonella Giannantoni, Marilena Gubbiotti, Naoki Yoshimura, and Karl-Erik Andersson

20 **Intravesical Therapy of Interstitial Cystitis** 95
Philip Hanno

21 **Botulinum Toxin in Treatment of Bladder Pain Syndrome/Interstitial Cystitis** 101
Paulo Dinis

22 **Intravesical Therapy and Its Evolution Over Three Decades, A European View** 105
Mauro Cervigni

23 **The Use of Heparin** 111
Arndt van Ophoven

24 **What Happened to Eosinophilic Cationic Protein: A Dead End** 113
Philip Hanno

25 **The Use of Pentosan Polysulfate in the Management of Interstitial Cystitis** 115
Robert M. Moldwin

26 **Etiology of Interstitial Cystitis and the Role of Pentosanpolysulfate in IC Therapy** 121
C. Lowell Parsons

27 Use of Transcutaneous Electrical Nerve Stimulation in the Management of Bladder Pain Syndrome 127
Magnus Fall

28 Use of Transcutaneous Electrical Nerve Stimulation in the Management of Bladder Pain Syndrome: 2017 Update 131
Kenneth M. Peters

29 Reappraisal of Transurethral Resection in Classic Interstitial Cystitis 135
Magnus Fall

30 Treatment of Interstitial Cystitis with the Neodymium YAG Laser: A Swedish View 139
Magnus Fall

31 Treatment of Interstitial Cystitis with the Neodymium YAG Laser: The Russian View 141
Andrew Zaitcev

32 Partial Denervation Procedures for Bladder Pain Syndrome 143
Rajesh Taneja

33 Surgical Therapy of Bladder Pain Syndrome 145
Tomohiro Ueda, Jørgen Nordling, Ralph Peeker, and Magnus Fall

34 The Birth of Conservative Management, Prescription Drug Applications, and Pelvic Floor Physical Therapy 149
Rebecca Rinko, Nima Shah, Melissa Dawson, and Kristene Whitmore

35 Placing Interstitial Cystitis/Bladder Pain Syndrome on the Map: The Story of the Interstitial Cystitis Association 155
Vicki Ratner

36 Back to the Future: Looking Forward by Examining the Past 161
John W. Kusek and Chris Mullins

37 Afterword 165
Philip Hanno and Alan Wein

Addendum 1: International Consultation 167

Addendum 2: AUA Guideline 173

Addendum 3: Asian Algorithm 175

Introduction

1

Philip Hanno, David Staskin, Alan Wein,
Jørgen Nordling, and Jean Jacques Wyndaele

Dr. Guy LeRoy Hunner, 1868–1957, a Johns Hopkins gynecologist, in a paper delivered to the Boston Medical Society described the 'Hunners Ulcer' in 1915. Seventy years later, in 1985 the idea of bringing together experts in the field of interstitial cystitis led to an assemblage following the 1986 International Continence Society meeting in Boston. This meeting was a unique opportunity to take advantage of the attendance and willingness of most of the authors who were internationally recognized in the field, and who eventually contributed to the first edition published in 1990.

Twenty-seven years is a long time between editions. Much has changed. Books and journals are no longer on library shelves, but exist in the ether. Much has not changed. Only two drugs are approved by the Food and Drug administration to treat IC/BPS, both of which were available when the first edition was printed. We think it is time to take a look back at how the field has advanced given the millions of dollars in research that have been devoted to it and the world-wide interest in the disorder that propelled the prevalence data from an estimated 40/100,000 to a current estimate of greater than 2700/100,000. What have we learned in the last 30 years, where are we now, and how can we best advance the field forward?

One hundred years after Hunner's paper, this text is intended to serve as an update of the first edition of *Interstitial Cystitis*, and to be of value to the researcher, clinician, and patient who seek a perspective as to where we are and how we got there. The format was chosen intentionally, as the majority of chapters take the unique approach of revisiting and revising and critiquing the initial text—"what we got right", "what we got wrong", "have we made progress?", and "in which direction should we should go?". Broad philosophical changes in approach to the patient and specific definitions; treatment algorithms for diagnosis and therapy; and basic science and clinical research into etiology and pharmacological

P. Hanno (✉)
Stanford University School of Medicine,
Stanford, CA, USA
e-mail: pmhanno@stanford.edu

D. Staskin
St. Elizabeth's Medical Center, Tufts University
School of Medicine, Boston, MA, USA
e-mail: staskinatt@gmail.com

A. Wein
Penn Medicine, Perelman School of Medicine,
Perelman Center for Advanced Medicine,
University of Pennsylvania Health System,
Philadelphia, PA, USA
e-mail: Alan.wein@uphs.upenn.edu

J. Nordling
Department of Urology, Herlev Hospital,
Herlev, Denmark
e-mail: jnordling@dadlnet.dk

J.J. Wyndaele
Department of Urology, Antwerp University, GGW,
Wilrijk, Antwerp, Belgium
e-mail: wyndaelejj@skynet.be

P.M. Hanno et al. (eds.), *Bladder Pain Syndrome – An Evolution*,
https://doi.org/10.1007/978-3-319-61449-6_1

therapy have all contributed to a new 'state of the art'. But, how much have we progressed? Was Hunner's description of an 'elusive ulcer' a prelude to the current understanding of chronic pelvic pain syndromes and the components? We will reserve judgment to the reader.

This book builds upon the knowledge base of the first edition. New commentary by some of the same authors and the addition of younger experts gives a balanced view of the field. There is no attempt to synthesize a single view of the controversial aspects of bladder pain syndrome, but rather we include many opinions and let the readers decide for themselves. Where possible, authors highlight the seminal publications that guided their thinking. The book concludes with up to date guidelines and management suggestions that provide a quick-reference for healthcare providers.

We would like to thank the authors for their expertise and dedication to this project. We want to thank the members of the International Association for the Study of Bladder Pain Syndrome (ESSIC), many of whom contributed to this volume, for their dedication directed at helping patients suffering from bladder pain syndrome. We all owe tremendous gratitude to the patients and patient groups that have also helped to expand the knowledge base aimed at alleviating the terrible symptoms associated with BPS and helping to find cures. We hope that the next edition planned for 2045 will treat bladder pain syndrome and interstitial cystitis as recognizable diseases with straightforward cures. We take pause to remember Robert Krane, M.D., our colleague who was a co-editor of the first edition.

2 Historical Perspectives

Jane Meijlink

2.1 Bladder Pain Syndrome … 30 Years Later

Enigmatic painful bladders and mysterious "ulcers" in the urinary bladder first appeared in medical publications in the early nineteenth century. Medical textbooks at the time drew a clear distinction between bladder neuralgia and bladder ulcers or lesions. However, by the beginning of the twentieth century, increasing use of the cystoscope may have led surgeons to focus on visible pathology, including ulcers and lesions, to the neglect of bladder neuralgia with invisible causes. Furthermore, Freudian theories prevalent at that period claiming women were "more prone to neurosis and hysteria" would have led to many women with urogenital pain being dismissed as psychosomatic and hysterical. While the original eighteenth to nineteenth century term "neurosis" referred to a neurological disorder, Freud's version of neurosis inferred a psychological/hysterical disorder as used by Walsh in this book. This has regrettably been a cause of great harm to women and their health, particularly in urogenital fields, and has not entirely disappeared today.

In the nineteenth century, as noted by Walsh, "interstitial cystitis" was a term used to describe a non-specific pathologic condition with inflammation in interstitial tissue caused by many diseases, disorders or trauma. The first mention of this term (found so far) was by Samuel D. Gross in 1876. In Germany, however, Maximilian Nitze was writing about a bladder disorder with frequency, pain and inflammatory ulceration of the mucosa which he described as "cystitis parenchymatosa", a term which was not to survive, but which was, however, used by Howard Kelly in 1898 to describe "when inflammation extends into the muscular vesical wall".

2.2 Howard Atwood Kelly (1858–1943): Pioneer in the Irritable Bladder

The Johns Hopkins Hospital in Baltimore, opened in 1889, was a centre of excellence in the United States. Howard Kelly, head of the new gynaecology and obstetrics department and Guy Hunner's boss, had a special interest in female urology and this laid the foundation for Guy Hunner's work with patients with a painful bladder. Howard Kelly, who had travelled extensively in Europe, took the Nitze cystoscope back to the Johns Hopkins Hospital in Baltimore and developed his own air distension version. Kelly had an interest in what he termed the irritable bladder: "A differential diagnosis must be made between cystitis and an irritable bladder or a hyperemia of the trigonum. In an 'irritable

J. Meijlink
International Painful Bladder Foundation,
Naarden, The Netherlands
e-mail: jane-m@dds.nl

P.M. Hanno et al. (eds.), *Bladder Pain Syndrome – An Evolution*,
https://doi.org/10.1007/978-3-319-61449-6_2

bladder' there is no inflammation and there is no pus in the urine, and no inflammatory area is seen," he wrote in 1922. He further noted that "the condition is dependent as a rule upon abnormal sensibility of the nerves of the bladder either at their ending or at some point in their course. With this anatomical basis a number of conditions bring about the disturbance which would not cause it in a healthy adult". With regard to treatment, he recommended that "where the central nervous system is involved, the treatment should be directed towards this." This was remarkably forward thinking at the time, bearing in mind that it is only in recent years that researchers have been investigating the "new" concept of central sensitization. Like others, Kelly had already discovered that "such items of diet as tomatoes, fruits, or acids, should be avoided when the patient finds that they aggravate her condition".

2.3 Guy Leroy Hunner (1868–1957): Bladder Ulcers and Lesions

When Guy Hunner joined Howard Kelly's department, he consequently had every opportunity to study urological as well as gynaecological disorders in women. In 1899, Hunner was given leave by Kelly for a 4-month study visit to Europe to familiarize himself with the latest medical knowledge and insights. Endoscopy was now rapidly becoming all the rage in Europe, with the cystoscope opening up new horizons in urology. Eminent surgeons, including Hurry Fenwick in London, had published papers on perforating ulcers and simple solitary ulcers of unknown cause and this may have caught the interest of Guy Hunner. However, Hunner felt that most of the ulcers he was seeing differed from Fenwick's simple solitary ulcers. Guy Hunner was the first person to publish a detailed report about painful bladders and to describe what he saw through the cystoscope, case by case. Since by 1930 Hunner wrote that he now had over 200 patients, he was considered the expert in this field in the United States. While he concentrated on ulcer and lesion pathology, Hunner did not forget patients with pain, urgency and frequency in whom the inside of the bladder appeared normal. His papers of 1915 and 1918 were seen as the "guideline" for many decades and consulted extensively. This is probably the reason why the term Hunner's ulcer was passed down from generation to generation. Hunner reported in 1918 that his colleague Dr. Cullen had suggested the name "elusive ulcer" due to the difficulty in locating the ulcer part of the lesion, but in his own opinion "it fails to describe adequately the widespread character of the chronic inflammatory involvement of the bladder walls."

Walsh is of the opinion that Hunner's use of the term "ulcer" led people to think that the disease might be focal. However, Hunner himself did not think it was focal but widespread, as we have seen above. Hunner also made a clear distinction in his publications between lesions and ulcers. Since his study of more than 200 of these patients took place over a period of at least 20 years, during which time cystoscopes would have been continually improving, it is debatable whether his belief that he was seeing true ulcers was entirely due to poor vision from the cystoscope. However, any meaningful comparison between Hunner's time and the situation today is always going to be problematic since he worked in an era when disease, infection and trauma were rife, antibiotics had not yet been invented, and women were very prudish and would probably have waited a very long time before plucking up the courage to consult a physician and may have concealed some of the more embarrassing details.

However, there is little doubt that his widely consulted publications did result in generations of urologists looking specifically for true ulcers and it could also be conjectured that the resultant focus on ulcers and lesions may have contributed to subsequent neglect of the non-lesion group—the *tic douloureux*—for many years.

2.4 John R. Hand

A new milestone was achieved in 1949 when John R. Hand from the Portland Clinic published a detailed, comprehensive study (223 patients: 204 women, 19 men) and literature review of what he now called "interstitial cystitis", noting "I am inclined to agree with Folsom's pithy comment that when Hunner 'delivered this child into the urologic world he did not name it as well as he described it'." Hand felt that "until a better name is found, "interstitial cystitis" is the most suitable since it is the only name with sufficient latitude to cover a diagnosis of the early as well as the late stages of the process." A year later, Seaman writes that the "term "interstitial cystitis" seems to epitomize the pathological picture better than the 14 other names by which it has been designated and which seem only to confuse the issue." We now therefore see that "interstitial cystitis" has moved away from being simply a pathology and has become the name of a painful bladder disease with "lesions".

Hand presented a grading system for lesions, subdivided into three grades. There was, however, no mention of "ulcers" and no reference to non-lesion painful bladders. He noted that some of their patients had now been treated with antibacterial sulfonamides introduced in the 1930s and that the new pioneering antibiotic penicillin had been tried on three patients.

When performing cystoscopy, Hand recommended that the bladder should be distended, emptied and distended a second time in order to avoid overlooking the early lesions of interstitial cystitis. He noted that on distention small discrete submucosal hemorrhages and dotlike bleeding points could be observed.

While numerous theories had been put forward concerning etiology, Hand was inclined to believe that interstitial cystitis is caused by a neurogenic factor. The proliferation of nerve tissue mentioned by Hand also caught the attention of Walsh.

Hand drew attention to comorbidities in these patients, noting that "allergies were more common among the patients with interstitial cystitis than among those from the general admission." He also reported that Fister drew attention to the striking similarity of some features of interstitial cystitis and Lupus erythematosus.

Like others before him, Hand noted that there is a large element of individual variation in these patients.

2.5 Campbell's Urology 1978: "An Irritable Bladder in an Irritable Patient"

Interstitial cystitis received a huge boost in awareness when Anthony Walsh was invited to write Chap. 19 on Interstitial Cystitis for the 1978 edition of Campbell's Urology where he famously described "an irritable bladder in an irritable patient". Here too he notes that "the synonym 'Hunner's Ulcer' has led many less experienced physicians to expect to see an ulcer at cystoscopy, and when no ulcer could be found, they erroneously failed to diagnose many genuine cases." True ulceration is rarely seen, noted Walsh. In recent years, lesion expert Magnus Fall has described the Hunner's Ulcer as a "vulnus" or wound seen only upon distension.

The tiny, punctate red dots seen after distension are "an experience that we describe as glomerulation". However, he emphasized that glomerulation is not absolutely pathognomonic, since it has been seen after distension in patients with dyskinesia.

Despite Walsh's warnings, the term Hunner's ulcer continued to be used and to mislead, while glomerulation was adopted as a hallmark of interstitial cystitis and incorporated into criteria.

Until this point, patients with no lesions were considered to have an early stage of the lesion disease. However, in 1978 Messing and Stamey pointed out that "we have no direct evidence that the classic disease will eventually develop in patients in the early group".

This was further reinforced in 1987 when Fall et al., describing interstitial cystitis as a heterogeneous syndrome, reported that they had observed clear differences between lesion and non-lesion disease which they considered to be two separate conditions and which, they emphasized, should be studied separately in clinical studies. This advice was unfortunately also largely ignored with a mixed bag of patients still participating in clinical studies and drug trials, rendering all results very questionable for years to come.

2.6 Interstitial Cystitis Association and the NIDDK

A major impulse was the founding of the Interstitial Cystitis Association (ICA) in 1984 in the United States by Dr. Vicki Ratner, an IC patient and orthopaedic surgeon. The ICA's success in sparking the interest of the National Institute of Diabetes and Digestive and Kidney Diseases (NIDDK) led to more coordinated research, an attempt to define the disease and the creation of strict diagnostic criteria for research purposes in 1987 at a workshop and later published in 1988. However, it was soon clear that the criteria needed to be modified since there was a risk of 20–40% of patients diagnosed with IC now being excluded. The revised criteria were published in the 1990 first edition of this book but not in a journal, resulting in many physicians being unaware of them. The 1987 criteria therefore continued to be used extensively worldwide including for clinical diagnosis which had never been the intention.

The Interstitial Cystitis Data Base (ICDB) Study eligibility criteria which were less stringent did not stipulate mandatory cystoscopy for participating patients. Consequently, once again no distinction was made between patients with or without Hunner lesions in studies.

By 1999 it was clear, according to Hanno et al., that strict application of NIDDK criteria would have misdiagnosed some 60% of patients believed by clinicians to have some form of interstitial cystitis, although by this time it was starting to become somewhat unclear exactly what was meant by interstitial cystitis.

As the new millennium dawned, it was becoming evident that consensus was lacking between different parts of the world, with the USA interpreting the term IC more freely—to the extent that it could by no means be called a rare disease in the US—while the rest of the world was still following the more restricted interpretation of the NIDDK criteria. Whereas the NIDDK had previously been seen as the IC Oracle of Delphi, research was now going global with greatly increasing interest in East Asia focusing around Japan where the Society of Interstitial Cystitis of Japan (SICJ) was set up, followed by an East Asian (Japan, South Korea, Taiwan) IC study group. An international conference—ICICJ—organised in Japan in 2003 revealed many of the cultural and scientific differences which were hindering further progress. Shortly afterwards, a European IC scientific meeting was held and ESSIC was set up.

2.7 Standards and Guidelines

In its 2002 Standardization of Lower Urinary Tract Function, the International Continence Society (ICS) Standardisation Committee reserved the name IC for a specific diagnosis based on typical cystoscopic and histological features (unfortunately without clearly specifying these features), while using "painful bladder syndrome (PBS)" for patients with symptoms but no identifiable infection or pathology. Since this was rather unclear to many people, the name simply became IC/PBS or PBS/IC while study or drug trial patients continued to be a mixture of both lesion and non-lesion.

Sparks were soon to fly when ESSIC published Diagnostic Criteria, Classification, and Nomenclature for Painful Bladder Syndrome/Interstitial Cystitis: An ESSIC Proposal, but soon decided to abolish the name IC altogether and henceforth use the name "bladder pain syndrome", as they announced at an NIDDK conference held in 2006. There was an uproar, including from the now extensive international IC patient movement which had not been consulted on any of the name changes. Nobody had taken into consideration any potential impact on the patients of a name change with respect to licensing issues and reimbursement, or eligibility for social security and disability allowances. The new name did not go down too well in East Asia either where they felt that it excluded patients who felt bladder pressure or discomfort but not what the patient interpreted as pain. This led to the revival of an old ICS term "hypersensitive bladder" in East Asia. Hypersensitive bladder symptoms consist of either pain or pressure or discomfort in the bladder usually with urinary frequency day and night and an urgent need to void. In the East Asian IC study group's Hypersensitive Bladder (HSB) concept, HSB and non-lesion IC are hypersensitive bladder disorders while Hunner lesion IC is an immuno-inflammatory disease. This study group believes that patients should not be treated as a single entity simply because they have similar symptoms.

Within the space of a decade, a flurry of diagnostic and treatment guidelines and standardisation documents appeared, none precisely the same, and some so long and convoluted as to be unreadable by the everyday urologist, let alone primary care. These included the European Association of Urology's Chronic Pelvic Pain Guideline, The American Urological Association IC/BPS Guideline, more recently the United Kingdom Joint RCOG/BSUG Guideline on Management of Bladder Pain Syndrome which included a focus on primary care, the ICS Standard for Terminology in Chronic Pelvic Pain Syndromes, Japanese and East Asian guidelines on IC and hypersensitive bladder and the Chronic Pelvic Pain Syndromes taxonomy by the International Association for the Study of Pain (IASP), as well as papers published by the French Nantes research group on pelvic visceral hypersensitivity.

Despite many articles since 1978 warning that glomerulation was not a reliable criterion, no further action was taken until the publication of a review paper by Wennevik et al. on the role of glomerulations in bladder pain syndrome. This concluded that there is no convincing evidence in the reviewed literature that glomerulations should be included in the diagnosis or phenotyping of bladder pain syndrome/interstitial cystitis and that glomerulations do not correlate with symptoms and are found in patients without bladder pain syndrome/interstitial cystitis. However, the East Asian IC study group announced that it would be continuing to record which patients develop what they term "mucosal bleeding after distension" (MBAD), but point out in their 2015 guideline update that MBAD and glomerulations are not identical. MBAD is bleeding from the bladder mucosa during drainage, while glomerulations are pinpoint haemorrhagic lesions or petechiae.

2.8 NIDDK MAPP Research Network

In 2008, the NIDDK, uncomfortably aware that expensive research in the past had produced no benefits for the patients, now opted for a different, wider approach when it launched its Multidisciplinary Approach to the Study of Chronic Pelvic Pain (MAPP) research network project, aimed at gaining a better understanding of both interstitial cystitis/ bladder pain syndrome (IC/BPS) and chronic prostatitis/chronic pelvic pain syndrome (CP/CPPS), now embracing a systemic—or whole-body—approach, investigating potential relationships between these conditions and other chronic conditions that are sometimes seen in IC/BPS and CP/CPPS patients, such as irritable bowel syndrome, fibromyalgia, and chronic fatigue syndrome. However, in phase I the MAPP research also failed to draw a distinction in its studies between lesion and non-lesion. This was remedied in phase II. A prominent role is now being played by research into phenotyping with the aim of sorting out the patients, currently bundled together. One aim is ultimately to find the most appropriate treatment for each subtype.

2.9 Ketamine Cystitis

The development in recent years of bladder pain, urgency and frequency often combined with very severe lesions in street ketamine users has led to ongoing research worldwide into this phenomenon. This is being closely followed by the IC/BPS world in the hope that it may generate new insights into lesions and shed light on why some users develop ketamine cystitis while others do not.

2.10 Basis for Research Is Consensus

The basis for meaningful research must be international consensus on nomenclature, definitions and criteria, while allowing for flexibility for clinical purposes, with all stakeholders involved including patient organisations since they are an invaluable source of knowledge about the full spectrum of patients and the impact in practical terms. [TAU] This consensus must therefore be an important goal.

2.11 Awareness and Information

Thanks to the drive by both medical societies and patient organisations there is now more awareness of not only IC/BPS and its comorbidities, but also of the sexual, social and emotional impact of the disease on the patient. Many books have been published for both patients and the medical world while the advent of the Internet has opened up a vast store of electronic information that Walsh could never have envisaged.

However, with urology societies tending to focus increasingly on oncology and male problems, it is essential to get more information and guidance out to (uro)gynaecologists. Today, with all physicians faced with less time and more patients, guidelines must be succinct and freely accessible online for quick and easy reference and importantly include information for primary care. Urologists and urogynaecologists also need more information about comorbidities so as to know when and to whom to refer their IC/BPS patients. A multidisciplinary approach is crucial for patients with IC/BPS and comorbidities.

2.12 Treatment: Right Treatment for Right Patient

Since Hunner's time, every imaginable treatment has been tried, many based on different theories. It has been estimated that over 180 treatments have been tried so far, a clear indication that something is very wrong. Everything works in a few patients, nothing is effective in all. Treatment is therefore highly individual.

Lesions are proving easier to treat than non-lesion bladders so these must be diagnosed at the earliest possible stage. To facilitate this, a comprehensive atlas of lesions would be of great value.

It is the large group of non-lesion IC/BPS patients which now urgently needs phenotyping so as to find the *right treatment for the right patient* at the earliest possible stage.

Above it, it should be remembered that a bladder disease like IC/BPS with pain, urgency and frequency can turn a normal person into an anxious, stressed, depressed recluse. Therefore, as Guy Hunner was fully aware, an important part of treatment for all patients is empathy and understanding.

Bibliography

1. Abrams P, Blaivas JG, Stanton S, Andersen JT. The standardisation of terminology of lower urinary tract function. The International Continence Society Committee on standardisation of terminology. Neurourol Urodyn. 1988;7:403–26.
2. Baranowski AP, Berger R, Buffington T, Collett B, Emmanuel A, Fall M, Hanno P, Howard F, Hughes J, Nickel JC, Nordling J, Tripp D, Vincent K, Wesselmann U, Williams AC. International Association for the Study of Pain (IASP) classification of chronic pain. Descriptions of chronic pain syndromes and definitions of pain terms. 2nd ed.; 2011. http://www.iasp-pain.org/files/Content/ContentFolders/Publications2/ClassificationofChronicPain/Part_II-F.pdf. Accessed 24 Jan 2017.

3. Doggweiler R, Whitmore KE, Meijlink JM, Drake MJ, Frawley H, Nordling J, Hanno P, Fraser MO, Homma Y, Garrido G, Gomes MJ, Elneil S, van de Merwe JP, Lin AT, Tomoe H. A standard for terminology in chronic pelvic pain syndromes: a report from the chronic pelvic pain working group of the international continence society. Neurourol Urodyn. 2017;36(4):984–1008. doi:10.1002/nau.23072.
4. Engeler D, Baranowski AP, Borovicka J, Cottrell A, Dinis-Oliveira P, Elneil S, Hughes J, Messelink EJ, Van Ophoven A, Reisman Y, Williams AC de C. Guidelines on chronic pelvic pain. Eur Assoc Urol. 2014. https://uroweb.org/wp-content/uploads/26-Chronic-Pelvic-Pain_LR.pdf. Accessed 24 Jan 2017.
5. Fall M, Johansson SL, Aldenborg F. Chronic interstitial cystitis: a heterogeneous syndrome. J Urol. 1987;137:35–8.
6. Fister GM. Similarity of interstitial cystitis (Hunner ulcer) to lupus erythematosus. J Urol. 1938;40:37.
7. Gillenwater JY, Wein AJ. Summary of the National Institute of arthritis, diabetes, digestive and kidney diseases. Workshop on interstitial cystitis, National Institutes of Health, Bethesda, Maryland, August 28–29, 1987. J Urol. 1988;140:203–6.
8. Gross SD. In: Gross SW, editor. A practical treatise on the diseases, injuries and malformations of the urinary bladder, the prostate gland and the urethra. 3rd ed. Philadelphia: Henry C. Lea; 1976.
9. Hand JR. Interstitial cystitis: report of 223 cases (204 women and 19 men). J Urol. 1949;61(2):291–310.
10. Hanno PM, Burks DA, Clemens JQ, Dmochowski RR, Erickson D, FitzGerald MP, Forrest JB, Gordon B, Gray M, Mayer RD, Moldwin R, Newman DK, Nyberg Jr L, Payne CK, Wesselmann U, Faraday MM. American Urological Association. Diagnosis and treatment of interstitial cystitis/bladder pain syndrome. 2014. http://www.auanet.org/education/guidelines/ic-bladder-pain-syndrome.cfm. Accessed 24 Jan 2017.
11. Hanno PM, Landis JR, Matthews-Cook Y, Kusek J, Nyberg L. The diagnosis of interstitial cystitis revisited: lessons learned from the National Institute of Health Interstitial Cystitis Database Study. J Urol. 1999;161:553–7.
12. Homma Y, Ueda T, Tomoe H, Lin AT, Kuo HC, Lee MH, SJ O, Kim JC, Lee KS. Clinical guidelines for interstitial cystitis and hypersensitive bladder updated in 2015. Int J Urol. 2016;23(7):542–9. doi:10.1111/iju.13118.
13. Homma Y, Ueda T, Tomoe H, et al. Clinical guidelines for interstitial cystitis and hypersensitive bladder syndrome. The Interstitial Cystitis Guideline Committee. Int J Urol. 2009;16:597–615.
14. Homma Y, Ueda T, Tomoe H, Lin AT, Kuo HC, Lee MH, SJ O, Kim JC, Lee KS. Clinical guidelines for interstitial cystitis and hypersensitive bladder updated in 2015. Int J Urol. 2016;23(7):542–9.
15. Hunner GL. A rare type of bladder ulcer in women; report of cases. Boston Med Surg J. 1915;172:660–4. Tr. South. Surg. Gynec. Assoc., 1914, 27
16. Hunner GL. Elusive ulcer of the bladder: further notes on a rare type of bladder ulcer with a report of twenty-five cases. Am J Obstet Dis Child. 1918;78:3–8.
17. Hunner GL. Letter to Dr Alan Chesney, June 30, 1947. Alan Mason Chesney Medical Archives.
18. Hunner GL. Neurosis of the bladder. J Urol. 1930;24:567–85.
19. Kelly HA. Operative gynaecology, vol. 1. New York: D. Appleton & Company; 1898.
20. Kelly HA, Burnham CF. Diseases of the kidneys, ureters and bladder, vol. 2. New York: D. Appleton & Company; 1922.
21. Kelly HA. Operative gynecology, vol. 1. 2nd ed. New York: D. Appleton & Company; 1912.
22. Meijlink JM, Kerrebroeck P. Chapter 28: interstitial cystitis: from Enigma to International Consensus. In: Felderhof E, Mattelaer J, Moll F, Schultheiss D, Van Kerrebroeck P, editors. Milestones in urology: EAU History Office and Davidsfond Uitgeverij NV; 2015.
23. Meijlink JM, Moldwin RM. The evolution of therapy for chronic pelvic pain. In: Moldwin RM, editor. Urological and gynaecological chronic pelvic pain. Cham: Springer; 2017. doi:10.1007/978-3-319-48464-8_1.
24. Meijlink JM. Interstitial cystitis and the painful bladder: a brief history of nomenclature, definitions and criteria. Int J Urol. 2014;21(Suppl 1):4–12. doi:10.1111/iju.12307.
25. Meijlink JM. Patient-centred standardization in interstitial cystitis/bladder pain syndrome—a PLEA. Transl Androl Urol. 2015;4(5):499–505. doi:10.3978/j.issn.2223-4683.2015.08.02.
26. Messing EM, Stamey TA. Interstitial cystitis: early diagnosis, pathology, and treatment. Urology. 1978;12:381–92.
27. Nitze M. Lehrbuch der Zystoskopie: Ihre Technik und Klinische Bedeutung. Berlin: JE Bergman; 1907. p. 410.
28. Nordling J, Wyndaele JJ, van de Merwe JP, Bouchelouche P, Cervigni M, Fall M. Bladder pain syndrome, a guide for clinicians. Springer; 2013. ISBN: 978-1-4419-6928-6.
29. Gross SD. A practical treatise on the diseases, injuries and malformations of the urinary bladder, the prostate gland and the urethra, 3rd ed. (Revised and Edited by Gross SW). Philadelphia: Henry C. Lea; 1976.
30. Seaman JA. Interstitial cystitis. J Urol. 1950;63(1):105–15. PMID: 15400266
31. Simon LJ, Landis JR, Erickson DR, Nyberg LM. The interstitial cystitis data base study: concepts and preliminary baseline descriptive statistics. Urology. 1997;49(5A Suppl):64–75.
32. Tirlapur SA, Birch JV, Carberry CL, Khan KS, Latthe PM, Jha S, Ward KL, Irving A. On behalf of the Royal College of obstetricians and gynaecologists. UK joint RCOG/BSUG guideline on management of bladder pain syndrome. BJOG. 2017;124(2):e46–72.

33. Walsh A. Interstitial cystitis. In: Harrison JH, editor. Campbell's urology. 4th ed. Philadelphia: WB Saunders; 1978. p. 693–707.
34. Van de Merwe JP, Nordling J, Bouchelouche P, et al. Diagnostic criteria, classification, and nomenclature for painful bladder syndrome/interstitial cystitis: an ESSIC proposal. Eur Urol. 2008;53:60–7.
35. Wennevik GE, Meijlink JM, Hanno P, Nordling J. The role of glomerulations in bladder pain syndrome—a review. J Urol. 2016;195(1):19–25.

3 The Epidemiology of Interstitial Cystitis/Bladder Pain Syndrome (IC/BPS): How Good Was a Study of 30-Years Ago

Philip J. Held, Philip Hanno, and Frank McCormick

Abbreviations

ACA	Affordable Care Act
CP/CPPS	Chronic prostatitis/Chronic pelvic pain syndrome
FDA	US Food and Drug Administration
Medicaid	A US Public Program that provides health insurance to the poor. this program is both Federal and State run
Medicare	The Public US Health Insurance Institution providing medical care to the elderly, disabled, end stage renal disease patients, and selected dependent groups
NIDDK	National Institute of Diabetes and Digestive Diseases and Kidney Diseases (NIDDK)
NIH	National Institutes of Health (there are 27 institutes)
ObamaCare	Another Name for the Affordable Care Act
QoL	Quality of life
RAND	Research and Development; A Private American Research Institution

P.J. Held, Ph.D. (✉)
Division of Nephrology, Stanford University, School of Medicine, Stanford, CA, USA
e-mail: esrd00@gmail.com

P. Hanno, M.D.
Stanford University School of Medicine, Stanford, CA, USA
e-mail: Philip.hanno@stanford.edu

F. McCormick, Ph.D.
Bank of America (Retired), Charlotte, NC, USA
e-mail: fmccorm@astound.net

3.1 Introduction

In 1987, Held, Hanno, Wein, Pauly, and Cahn (hereafter Held-Hanno) conducted an epidemiologic study of Interstitial Cystitis (IC) a rare project at the time. (Later published in 1990). The study was to a great extent a response to the relevant clinical experiences of Dr. Hanno, a University of Pennsylvania urologist who had had many interactions with Dr. Vicki Ratner, an orthopedic surgeon and IC patient, who had experienced a life changing prolonged terrible experience with this chronic disease. Consequently Dr. Ratner had become politically and media active, which lead to a brief, 3-h Sunday afternoon workshop at the suggestion of the NIH. This gathering financed and lead by Dr. Alan Wein, chair of Urology at Penn, brought in an economist, Dr. Held, who had a propensity to see the research world through empirical

P.M. Hanno et al. (eds.), *Bladder Pain Syndrome – An Evolution*, https://doi.org/10.1007/978-3-319-61449-6_3

data collection and analysis where his focus had been on end stage renal disease. Some time prior to this meeting, the NIH had requested eight noted urologists to write a short memo answering the question: what do you know about IC? Held's response on reading these memos was: these distinguished urologists do not agree on anything and besides no one has any data. That was the birth of this $35,000 study (Held-Hanno) funded by two small grants from the Urban Institute and NIDDK of the NIH.

This study (Held-Hanno) sparked many changes in the knowledge, research focus, and perception of IC/BPS. One of the first major findings was IC/BPS was not, as had been reported in a basic urology text book:

> ***"...a rare psychosomatic disorder which 'may represent the end stage of a bladder that has been made irritable by emotional disturbances...a pathway for the discharge of unconscious hatred.'"*** (Urology, [1])

Prevalence was shown by the Held-Hanno study to be at least twice the rate previously reported by one of the few widely cited and reputable papers on the topic [2] which focused on one city in Finland. (Curiously a recent review of Oravisto's paper revealed that his study was based on a review of hospital records, which would likely have biased any measurements of prevalence to the low side).

Thirty years have passed since the publication of the Held-Hanno study. This short paper is intended to be a look back and look forward of what the substantial research on Interstitial Cystitis/ Bladder Pain Syndrome has determined. A quick assessment of the past thirty years research leads to one very strong conclusion:

Despite years of effort and millions of dollars of research, the status of things in the words of Persu et al. [3]:

> ***...because the pathological processes underlying the condition are not yet elucidated, biological markers of the condition are not yet available, and the type and severity of symptoms can vary, so, clearly defining the condition is not yet possible...***

This does not mean that the research was not worthwhile or that more research would be ill advised. In fact, quite the contrary, the problems are now known to be even larger, more demanding, and yes, still unanswered.

A tremendous amount of good epidemiologic research has been conducted and reported, from which two observations stand out:

1. All prevalence indicators show that whatever this IC/BPS is, it is not a rare disease and most likely is a chronic aliment that affects millions of Americans of both sexes but more dominantly women. Based on the research, IC/BPS is a very large public health problem that burdens many patients and deserves the research money focused on this chronic disease.
2. Apparently, epidemiologists think their professional duties do not merit or allow focusing on the economic implications of IC/BPS. Most of the epidemiology reported in this past period (1987–2017) did not even touch the economic issues while a few made a minor feint in that direction. Perhaps NIH, which funded most of these research projects, gave direct or subtle signals that economics was not of interest. But one should remember that the NIH is part of the US Public Health Service. In America today, it is hard to conceive, that projects doing research focused on such a costly heavy burdened disease did not think the cost, access to care, or the value of care did not merit more attention. We discuss economics and IC/BPS below at some length.

Perhaps the NIH has suggested that somehow economics of health care is not fitting to the pursing of the basics of health care in America. Some of this thinking points to presuming that Medicare, which has one of the largest budgets in the Federal Government (2016: $524B/year) should pay for health care while NIH ($31B) focuses exclusively on basic science. But Medicare's primary mission is to pay bills for medical care that hopefully NIH, via its focused research efforts, assures the public is efficient and good medical practice.

3.2 What Did This Early Study Tell Us? Has It Held Up Over Time?

Shown on the left side of Table 3.1 are ten points that capture the major findings of the 1987–1990 Held-Hanno study. The right side of Table 3.1 provides an answer yes or no whether the interim research has supported the original research and some brief notes on the interim research from this period.

Items 1 & 2. Prevalence, a central issue for study of any disease. Held-Hanno showed that the original study provided prevalence estimates that were far larger than the Finnish study. And clearly the right side of Table 3.1 indicates that practically all studies since have shown that prevalence is much higher than expected whether you use the baseline of Oravisto or Held-Hanno. As shown below (item 2), there was this ambiguity that occurred with the patient who experienced painful bladder and sterile urine but for whom there was no diagnosis of IC. So over this interim of 30 years, the evolution of thinking and classification of this disease resulted in combining the two notions into one IC/BPS.

But the right side of item 1 in Table 3.1 also identifies a major problem that has evolved from research and treatment of IC/BPS: there is considerable variance in these estimates especially if one includes the symptom studies. (e.g. Berry et all suggest there may be up to 7.9 million women in the US suffering from IC/S although only 10% have been given the diagnosis).

Items 3 & 4. While occurring in all ages, typically this disease occurs in middle age and the

"natural history of symptoms of IC … to be that of a sub acute onset with a rapid peak in severity,

Table 3.1 Interstitial cystitis/painful bladder syndrome: major findings of an early study (1987–1990) compared with current estimates

	Major findings from Held-Hanno 1987–1990[a]	Supported by subsequent research
1	43,500–90,000 diagnosed cases of IC in the USA (Almost twice the Finish (Oravisto) estimate of **18** vs. Held et al. of **30/100,000 women**)	Yes. All modern US estimates are higher than Held et al. including some as high as 7.9 M women.[b] Evolution of Nomenclature brought both IC and Bladder Pain Syndrome into one and the same disease: IC/BPS
2	Up to a fivefold increase in IC prevalence if all patients with painful bladder, sterile urine had been given the diagnosis, yielding up to half million possible cases in the USA	Yes; Definition has evolved to IC/BPS
3	Median age of onset: 40 years	Yes. E.g. Rand study: 45 years
4	Late deterioration in symptoms unusual	Yes
5	Ten times higher incidence of childhood bladder problems in IC patients vs. controls	Yes
6	Two times the incidence of a history of urinary tract infection vs. controls	Yes
7	Lower quality of life (QoL) than dialysis patients; Dyspareunia common.	Yes. All subsequent studies report low quality of life however using other comparison measures. E.g. "Lower in vitality and mental health". "IC had significantly lower QoL scores in four of the seven quality of life dimensions"[b]
8	Medical treatment cost: $13.9K/patient/yr. Lost economic production: $15.2K/patient/yr. (2017 prices)	Yes; but cursory at best Using Jones & Nyberg prevalence of 500/100K population: $47B total economic cost/yr
9	Treatments Frequently Ineffective	Yes. Still the case; Two treatments that sometimes help: pelvic floor physical therapy; diet modification
10	Unable to work outside the home	Yes, but comparison group not given

[a]Hanno [4]
[b]Berry et al. Symptom measure; women over 18 years; K=1,000, B=billion

and then a relatively constant plateau of chronic symptoms thereafter. However, many patients do experience …remissions and flares in their disease symptoms." [5]

Item 7. Quality of Life (QoL) The Held-Hanno study clearly showed that quality of life of IC/BPS patients was low and to make the measurement clear used a comparison group of patients living with chronic dialysis. All the subsequent studies, which addressed QoL, found much the same but provided comparisons that were not so obvious to benchmark.

Item 8. Costs were reported in many dimensions in the original study including estimates of medical care use (physician visits, hospital stays, insurance coverage and the like). Other cost measures included lost economic production attributed to IC/BPS because of lower labor force participation and lower wages when working in the labor force. Using the prevalence estimates of Jones and Nyberg (500/100,000 population) a projection of $47 billion economic cost per year including both medical care cost and lost economic production. However the studies in the interim had at best a weak focus on economics. In a section below we discuss at some length the significance of this omission.

Item 9. Treatments were frequently ineffective in the Held et al. study. And probably one of the most depressing news of this research arena is that the situation has not changed much since 1990. It is really depressing to report that there has been little progress in treating this chronic disease.

It has been 39 years since DMSO became the only FDA approved intravesical therapy for "interstitial cystitis", and 21 years since pentosan polysulfate became the only orally approved medication for this condition. While many newer therapies seem to have some benefit (neuromodulation, botulinum toxin, cyclosporine), none have made the threshold of FDA approval for this condition, and the vast majority of therapies are off-label. Perhaps the biggest advance has been in the use of pelvic floor physical therapy as a staple of a conservative treatment approach.

Item 10. Other important measures like the ability to hold employment were captured by Held-Hanno and importantly had comparison groups that were easy to interpret. Basically these IC/BPS patients are frequently out of the work force because of their disease. Unfortunately, the interim studies did not pursue these questions very well.

Overall the Held–Hanno study of 1990 performed remarkably well. Virtually all of the basic findings reported in 1990 have been confirmed and amplified in many cases in the following 30 years. Perhaps the only major issue that was not pursued in the early period, which came out of the subsequent studies, was the epidemiology of males with IC/BPS.

3.3 Prevalence of IC/BPS

Prevalence, usually expressed as # cases/population, is one of the most fundamental measurements of epidemiology. How many cases have this disease or this condition? Estimating the prevalence is an extremely important research component in understanding and coping with the IC/BPS medical condition. Prevalence indicates just how "big" a medical problem is as well as providing an indication of how the disease incidence (new cases per unit of time) and prevalence is changing. In the case of IC/BPS, Orivisto's 1975 study is generally considered an "original" if for no other reason than it was an early report. The study was based on a thorough examination of hospital records in one city in Finland in which was believed that all cases had a high likelihood of being counted. Four particular aspects of Oravisto estimates should be noted:

1. The cases were "determined" to be interstitial cystitis (IC);
2. Were diagnosed by a physician;
3. Were measured per population estimates of women.
4. Were based on a review of hospital records.

Subsequent work sometimes does and sometimes does not make these distinctions.

Prevalence estimate are important because:

1. The magnitude of the problem, in even the simplest terms, can be determined: e.g. "More than 1.2 million people in the US are living with HIV." But more quantitatively, prevalence

is the starting point for almost all policy questions. If you doubt this speak sometime to the physicians and patients involved in what are considered "rare diseases".

2. When combined with some measure of the cost of treatment (e.g. medical expenditures per patient per year) of a disease, it provides policy and decision makers with considerable information in determining priorities in allocation of research moneys. Or look into the pharmaceutical industry as they decide on putting a few billion dollars investment for a new product. Do you think they do not take seriously prevalence estimates? Not a total picture by any means but part of the picture. See below which discusses this topic in more detail.
3. As shown in Table 3.2, the National Institute of Diabetes, Digestive and Kidney Diseases (NIDDK one of 27 institutes and centers that make up the NIH) in 2016 spent almost 1.6 billion dollars ($1,563,393,000) on extramural research (about 86% of the total NIDDK budget of $1.9B). Just over a quarter (28%) of the extramural budget of NIDDK was spent on research focused on kidney, urological and hematological diseases. What fraction went to urological diseases including IC/BPS was not available.

The NIH/NIDDK decision process is clearly not a transparent function but one does not have to be a political genius to suppose that the social cost (money, quality of life, loss of life) of a disease plays a role in making decisions where to allocate extramural research funds. For example, in the case of renal failure, Medicare (the public institution in the US that "insures" the elderly, disabled and other categories of Americans) pays most of the bills for all dialysis and transplants regardless of age. But NIDDK puts a lot of research resources into the study of renal disease including end stage because it is very expensive in addition to being the cause of a lot of potentially preventable deaths. Politics plays a role too. Just look at the funding that went into the battles to treat AIDS.

Table 3.2 National Institutes of Health

National Institute of Diabetes and Digestive Diseases and Kidney Diseases (NIDDK)		
Extramural Research	2016 Fiscal Year	%
Diabetes, Endocrinology and Metabolic Diseases	$641,483,000	41
Digestive Diseases and Nutrition	$482,533,000	31
Kidney Urologic and Hematologic Diseases	$439,377,000	28
Subtotal, Extramural Research	$1,563,393,000	100

https://www.niddk.nih.gov/about-niddk/budget-legislative-information/Documents/National-Institute-of-Diabetes-and-Digestive-and-Kidney-Diseases-Fiscal-Year-2017-Budget_%20508.pdf. Total NIDDK budget is $1.82B

3.3.1 What the Held-Hanno and Subsequent Studies Tell US About Prevalence of IC/BPS

Essentially, the older study and most all US studies since confirm that IC/BPS is a serious health problem facing America. And given that the medical world has few helpful treatments, it is even a bigger problem than most. When there is medical technology (e.g. pharmaceuticals) and the problem might be financial access, the solution may be simple at least conceptually i.e. find the financing to fix the problem. (Interestingly the Konkle et al. [6] study gives a passing indication that a non-trivial number of the patients in the RAND study did not have health insurance).

Table 3.3 provides an overview of the prevalence findings of the Held-Hanno study and the subsequent research following in the period 1990–2016. Jones and Nyberg [5] suggest there are 1.1 million persons in the US with IC/BPS. Given that their study was based on a well-researched and respected data source (National Health Interview Survey), their estimates should be given additional credence. Suskin et al. 2013, a reasonably recent study, suggests that there are 2.1 M <u>men</u> with IC/BPS although they note that many of these cases may be currently diagnosed as having chronic pelvic pain syndrome/nonbacterial prostatitis.

Leppilahti et al. (2002–2005) used the O'Leary-Sant interstitial cystitis symptom and problem index (never validated for making a diagnosis per se) to select women with IC symptoms

Table 3.3 Prevalence of BPS/IC: 1990 vs. 2016 (rate per 100,000 population shown in bold)

Prevalence	Characteristics from Held-Hanno [7]	Current research/beliefs	Comment
Diagnosis based	2× Higher than Oravisto; 90,000 females, **30/**	All studies confirm that prevalence in US is much higher than Oravisto rate	All recent studies suggest this is a large public health problem
		E.G. Others:	
		Jones, Nyberg [5] **500/** ~ 1.1 million	
		Clemens [8] **197/** ~ 0.5 M	
		Suskin [9] ~ 2.1 M Men	
		Oleary Sant **100 to 300** 228–680 K	
Symptom based		Berry et al. **2700** Only 10% confirmed IC/BPS diagnosis	Berry suggests/3.3 To 7.9 M women >18 years of age with symptoms. 320–766 K with diagnosis of IC/BPS
Female to male ratio	Similar to Oravisto, 10/1	Maybe 5/1 or even more men than women, especially for symptom basis	Suskin: male cases likely include chronic prostatitis symptom (CPS)

from the Finnish population register. Of 1331 respondents, 32 had moderate or severe symptoms involving a suspicion of BPS/IC (symptom score 7 or higher). Of 21 who consented to clinical evaluation, 7 had probable or possible IC/BPS. Corrected estimates yielded a prevalence of 300 per 100,000 women [10, 11]. Similar studies without clinical confirmation suggested prevalence in Austrian women of 306/100,000 [12] and in Japanese women of 265/100,000 [13].

The highest and most recent prevalence estimates come from Berry et al. [14] which suggests an estimate of up to 7.9 million women over the age of 18 have symptoms consistent with IC/BPS. It is important to note that this estimate is based on symptoms not diagnoses. Berry et al. [14] also suggest that almost 10% of their prevalent symptom sample report a diagnosis of IC/BPS which translates to 320,000 to 760,000 women in the US.

Jones and Nyberg [5]:

> ***…It is unclear the extent to which these estimates represent true differences in prevalence, rather than reflect the different methods used to define an IC case…***

The evolution over the years of combining IC with BPS would be consistent with the Jones Nyberg [5] observation. The original Held-Hanno study reported similar results. It was reported, and somewhat of a surprise, that board certified urologists consistently reported that the number of patients with painful bladders and sterile urine far outnumbered the cases they had diagnosed as IC (Table 3.1, item 2 above).

Jones and Nyberg [5] continued with:

> ***…All studies of adults show a marked female predominance…***

Held-Hanno did not report on many cases of males, which suggests that the ratio reported by Oravisto of 10/1 female to male was generally consistent with this later study by Held-Hanno. However in the interim since this earlier Held-Hanno study, the Suskin et al. [9] report very large numbers of males with possible IC/BPS. But Suskin et al.'s estimates are likely to have included chronic prostatitis/chronic pelvic pain syndrome (CP/CPPS). In conclusion, the predominance of females in diagnosed IC/BPS may or may not be true as the research is ambiguous.

Basically many men have symptoms of BPS but have been diagnosed with CPPS, it is likely that anyone with symptoms of BPS has it if there is not a confusable disorder, and CPPS is not a confusable disorder being that it is a symptom complex itself. Granted they may overlap, but if you have BPS symptoms that meet the definition, you have BPS.

In conclusion, the Held-Hanno study certainly moved the ball off the tee as far as challenging the Oravisto estimate of prevalence. It is abundantly clear that both men and women report very high levels of IC/BPS symptoms compared to the Oravisto diagnosis rates. IC/BPS is no longer considered an extremely rare condition but the precise level of prevalence still has substantial variance. For research purposes however, it seems clear that more studies of prevalence are not warranted if the question is whether IC/BPS is a major public health problem. The answer is unquestionably yes.

3.3.2 How Well Did the Held-Hanno Paper Score on Prevalence?

The paper performed a service in opening up the discussions and research to the notion that IC/BPS was significantly under counted and diagnosed. The Held-Hanno finding that there were 5× as many PBS cases for each diagnosed IC patient was a real contribution. The Held-Hanno paper opened the doors to the notion that there were many, both women and men, with chronic painful non-bacterial bladder problems.

3.4 The Missing Case of Economics and Epidemiology

As has been argued above in Section I, measurement of economic parameters in the epidemiology of IC/BPS was a major contribution of the Held-Hanno paper of 1990. Correspondingly the absence of most any economics in the epidemiology since 1987 is a serious omission.

In Table 3.4 we lay out the case for measuring economic parameters in the study of IC/BPS. We make two general distinctions for including economics in the study or IC/BPS.

The first is the well recognized agenda of medical care use as measured by doctor visits, hospital stays, and pharmaceutics. There are of course other important resource use indicators that should be part of the overall picture of the treatment of IC/BPS such as nursing home, intermediate care facilities, durable medical goods and the like but the notion is clear that medical care finance is a major part of the care of the patient, the magnitude of the problem (combined with prevalence) and the priorities for funding research. Given the general ignorance level of basic science of IC/BPS as well as the clinical unknowns, the basic message for societal research objective is that this is a large public health problem deserving attention. Economics refines the discussion and quantifies the social message of treating, diagnosing, improving the patients' quality of life, and even curing the condition.

IC/BPS being a chronic painful disease with social integration problems (e.g. frequent voiding) is likely to produce labor force participation issues which lead to all sorts of other economic consequences including disability under the Social Security program and likely related medical insurance issues. Does the IC/BPS patient receive federal or state Disability benefits? This clearly represents a major quality of life issue besides pointing to the issues of who pays for this safety net, how prolonged, and how does recovery fit into this picture? (NIH is usually considered the relevant institution in researching IC/

Table 3.4 Most US Epidemiology Studies of IC/PBS in the past 30 years have had a very light focus on economics: a serious omission

A. Conventional & Routine $ Measures (e.g. Doctors, Hospital, Drugs, Insurance)	
1.	Combined with prevalence helps determine the social burden of IC/PBS
2.	A vital element to the setting of medical research priorities: to NIH; pharmaceutical companies; medical insurance
3.	Employment impediments are part of social cost and Quality of Life
4.	Disability payments tell a lot about patient well being & social cost
5.	Access & Impediments to Medical Care vital to patient well being
6.	Cost history might invoke pre-existing conditions issues with health insurance
B. Recent Research Advances Can Help to Determine Not only Cost but <u>Value</u> of Treatments and Cures	
1.	Imagine a measure of the social cost of IC/BPS
2.	Imagine what a signal as to what a cure is worth

BPS but if a substantial number of the patients with IC/BPS are receiving Disability benefits and corresponding Medicare insurance (not necessarily Medicare due to age) then Medicare may also be responsible for research in this arena. (Medicare plus 3 other public insurance programs (Medicaid, Children's Insurance, Affordable Care Act), represent approximately 25% of the total federal (2017) budget which combined with Social Security constitute over 50% of the Federal budget. As something of a control group consider that defense spending represents approximately 17%).

A large and constant public health issue in the US today (and for at least 50 years past) is health insurance: how accessible is it and for whom? How complete? What does it cost? Who pays? It is not that every epidemiology study of IC/BPS has to be an economic portrait of an IC/BPS patient, but there are some core areas of research that indicate much about the social burden of this disease. For example, Suskind et al. have an appendix, which has a few demographic and economic indicators:

The reported household income (2013) of Suskind's sample appears to be about $53,000 per year, which is just about the national average for that year. (https://www.google.com/webhp?sourceid=chromeinstant&rlz=1C5CHFA_enUS503US590&ion=1&espv=2&ie=UTF8#q=average+us+household+income+2013&).

Held-Hanno had a similar finding in their study for 1990.

In addition the Suskind sample has only 6.2% reporting that they did not have a high school degree when the US national average is approximately 12%. Both of these measures (household income and educational achievement) would suggest that IC/BPS is not a disease overly represented by the poor of America in contrast to a disease like diabetes or end stage renal disease.

However, these findings of typical household income levels raise all sorts of questions. At first glance typical household income would suggest these patients with IC/BPS may have more access to medical care than do the poor. This could be an explanation of possibly measured lower rates of IC/BPS among the poor rather than genuine biological true differences of IC/BPS. In other words measured rates of IC/BPS may depend on access to the medical system, which is why the recent epidemiology studies would have benefited by an economic component. Of course the epidemiologists are aware of such possible non-response bias and presumably took appropriate countermeasures. Whatever, it would be reassuring if the medical insurance status were measured. Similarly to the issue of household income and IC/BPS among the poor Suskind et al.'s appendix data suggest that Blacks (African American) are also underrepresented in their sampled population, again agreeing with the Held-Hanno study.

Curiously, Suskind et al. report that 38% of their sample (presumably males) were employed in the last month. While not an exact comparable statistic, the US Census reports that 70% of non institutionalized men in 2013 were employed (https://www.bls.gov/cps/aa2013/cpsaat02.pdf).

These men with IC/BPS have poor labor force participation which Held-Hanno reported for women in their 1990 study i.e. IC led many women to withdraw from the workforce because of their disease. Not only is this a serious economic/quality of life issue in itself, but also leads to another non-trivial issue of access to health insurance discussed above with regards to possible measurement bias of IC/BPS. The largest single source of health insurance in the US is employer group health insurance. For example over 70% of the non-elderly employed US population obtain their health insurance through an employer sponsored health insurance plan. While Medicaid (the US health insurance program for the poor) may cover 20% of the total, there is a non-trivial number of Americans who are basically without health insurance or have to purchase insurance on the "individual market" including those insured under the Affordable Care Act (Obamacare). So the issue of possible low employment in the labor force and the resultant conditions of obtaining health insurance has at least two implications for research focused on patients with IC/BPS:

1. Access to health insurance is likely reduced for these patients in this expensive American medical market compared to what patients

might consume if access was not an impediment. So researchers need to be focused on the issue of non-response bias if the counting of cases and diagnoses (prevalence) and subsequent outcomes start with access to medical care like physician visits. (A good question for Jones and Nyberg [5] is what did they do about possible non-response bias in their study based on the Health Interview Study?)

2. It may be a stretch given that currently many IC/BPS patients may not be diagnosed or treated. However if treatment and access to medical care are truly improved in the future for patients with IC/BPS, the chronic nature of this disease should alert the research community about "pre-existing conditions". This issue is in our news sources every day and is central to the design of any health insurance plan (both public and private), particularly in the individual market where persons outside the work force frequently find themselves. Briefly, if a patient's profile or history suggests they may present "high financial risk to the insurance plan, the incentive is there to not insure this person at or at least not at average premium rates. Think of auto insurance for young male drivers. They are a sure case of higher financial risk to insure which is why they are charged higher premiums. If an auto insurance company did not charge higher premiums for these high-risk drivers, the insurance company would lose clients of all ages as their premiums rise as a consequence of the high risk young males. The reason for concern for IC/BPS patients is that they may someday be identified as "high risk" and may have trouble buying health insurance.

While recent history with the issue has gained wide understanding in the body politic and passage of laws to prevent such conditions affecting insurance access, recent research focusing on Multiple Sclerosis (MS) patients, for example, has shown that insurance plans sometimes act on these adverse financial incentives in spite of the laws preventing such. (See [15]). There is one condition that may point in the treatment of patients with IC/BPS that would suggest these concerns about pre-existing conditions are over blown. Held-Hanno showed that IC/BPS patients may not be heavy users of inpatient hospital care, the widely recognized big driver of medical care cost. But this discussion is another indicator of information loss in the recent epidemiological studies ignoring all economic issues.

3.4.1 Determining Value of a Medical Intervention

Item B in Table 3.4 points to a very important new development in Health Services Research. Held, McCormick, Ojo, and Roberts published a paper in 2016 in the leading transplant journal (***American Journal of Transplantation***), which developed and applied new techniques to estimate the ***value*** of medical interventions and medical care. In this case they focused on the **benefits and value** of kidney transplantation and showed, for example, that the net societal value of a kidney transplant, after lifetime costs of $0.6 M, was approximately $1.9 M. The break through in this paper was the focus on **value**. Medical cost have been measured and published for some time. But putting value on medical interventions is relatively new and has many implications in allocating research funds, in signals to pharmaceutical industry, and in general deciding what the social injury of a medical problem is. The abstract of this Held and McCormick et al. paper is included in an Appendix. The entire paper can be downloaded free at: http://onlinelibrary.wiley.com/doi/10.1111/ajt.13490/full

The treatment of IC/BPS is certainly a long way off from the success of kidney transplantation. But this notion of estimating the value of treating a disease such as IC/BPS is certainly not impossible given the correct research objectives. For example, even under current conditions of poor treatment outcomes, if one were to measure the loss in the quality of life, the cost of current treatment methods one could reasonably estimate the social loss (negative value) that is borne by an IC/BPS patient. To estimate the total social value one would need estimates of prevalence, which we showed above to have considerable variance, but conservative estimates could be used to derive reasonable lower bound estimates. The result would be a quantified estimate of the total social burden of this disease. Such an estimate would be helpful in the debates for more research resources as shown above in Table 3.2.

Conclusion

This review of the comparisons and conclusions of the Held-Hanno [7] paper when compared to the IC/BPS research in the interim shows a very high success rate. The Held-Hanno paper established a number of hypotheses and observations that were subsequently confirmed by years and millions of dollars of research. The primary conclusions which were sparked by this earlier paper and have been supported by subsequent research include IC/BPS is:

1. A chronic major public health problem which is debilitating and frequently extremely painful with considerable degradations in the quality and functioning of life.
2. A disease whose treatment is frequently, if not generally unsuccessful if the goal is establishing a normal quality of life. This is the case in spite of tremendous investments of time and scarce resources. More is needed.
3. While the prevalence estimates have considerable variance IC/BPS is by no means a rare disease and likely include millions of Americans of both sexes.
4. Practically all the demographic measures of the IC/BPS patients originally reported by Held-Hanno, have been confirmed by the subsequent research of the last 30 years.

The socioeconomic issues laid out by Held-Hanno have not been researched by most all of the US epidemiological studies conducted in the last 30 years. This is most unfortunate since these issues are very important in determining vital issues in the treatment of this disease but particularly in the important task of providing a more complete picture of the social burden of this disease.

Appendix. A Cost-Benefit Analysis of Government Compensation of Kidney Donors*

P. J. Held, F. McCormick, A. Ojo, and J. P. Roberts

Abstract

From 5000 to 10,000 kidney patients die prematurely in the United States each year, and about 100,000 more suffer the debilitating effects of dialysis, because of a shortage of transplant kidneys. To reduce this shortage, many advocate having the government compensate kidney donors. This paper presents a comprehensive cost-benefit analysis of such a change. It considers not only the substantial savings to society because kidney recipients would no longer need expensive dialysis treatments—$1.45 million per kidney recipient—but also estimates the monetary value of the longer and healthier lives that kidney recipients enjoy—about $1.3million per recipient. These numbers dwarf the proposed $45,000-per-kidney compensation that might be needed to end the kidney shortage and eliminate the kidney transplant waiting list. From the viewpoint of society, the net benefit from saving thousands of lives each year and reducing the suffering of 100,000 more receiving dialysis would be about $46 billion per year, with the benefits exceeding the costs by a factor of 3. In addition, it would save taxpayers about $12 billion each year.

- *American Journal of Transplantation* 2015; XX: 1–9 Wiley Periodicals Inc. doi:10.1111/ajt.13490.

References

1. Walsh PC, Gittes RE, Perlmutter AD, Stamey TA, Saunders WB. Campbell's urology. 5th ed; 1986.
2. Oravisto KJ. Epidemiology of interstitial cystitis. Ann. Chir Gynaecol Fenn. 1975;64(2):75–7.
3. Persu C, Cauni V, Gutue S, Blaj I, Jinga V, Geavlete P. From interstitial cystitis to chronic pelvic pain. J Med Life. 2010;3(2):167–74.
4. Hanno PM. Interstitial cystitis—epidemiology, diagnostic criteria, clinical markers. Rev Urol. 2002;4(Suppl 1):S3–8.

5. Jones CA, Nyberg L. Epidemiology of interstitial cystitis. Urology. 1997;49(suppl 5A):2–9.
6. Konkle KS, Berry SH, Elliott MN, Hilton L, Suttorp MJ, Clauw DJ, Clemens JQ. Comparison of an interstitial cystitis/bladder pain syndrome clinical cohort with symptomatic community women from the RAND Interstitial Cystitis Epidemiology study. J Urol. 2012;187(2):508–12. doi:10.1016/j.juro.2011.10.040. Epub 2011 Dec 15
7. Held PJ, Hanno PM, Wein AJ, Pauly MV, Cahn MA. Chapter 4. Epidemiology of interstitial cystitis. In: Hanno PM, Staskin DR, Krane RJ, Wein AJ, editors. Interstitial cystitis. London: Springer; 1990. p. 29–48.
8. Clemens JQ, Meenan RT, O'Keeffe-Rosetti MC, et al. Prevalence of prostatitis-like symptoms in a managed care population. J Urol. 2006;176:593.
9. Suskind AM, Berry SH, Ewing BA, Elliott MN, Suttorp MJ, Clemens JQ. The prevalence and overlap of interstitial cystitis/bladder pain syndrome and chronic prostatitis/chronic pelvic pain syndrome in men; results of the RAND Interstitial Cystitis Epidemiology (RICE) male study. J Urol. 2013;189(1):141–5. doi:10.1016/j.juro.2012.08.088.
10. Lepiilahti TL, Tammela HH, Auvinen A. Prevalence of symptoms related to interstitial cystitis in women: a population based study in Finland. J Urol. 2002;168:139–43.
11. Leppilahti M, Sairanen J, Tammela TL, Aaltomaa S, Lehtoranta K, Auvinen A. Prevalence of clinically confirmed interstitial cystitis in women: a population based study in Finland. J Urol. 2005;174:581–3.
12. Temml C, Wehrberger C, Riedl C, Ponholzer A, Marszalek M, Madersbacher S. Prevalence and correlates for interstitial cystitis syptoms in women participating in a health-screening project. Eur Urol. 2007;51:803–8.
13. Inoue Y, Mita K, Kakehashi M, Kato M, Usiu T. Prevalence of painful bladder syndrome symptoms in adult women in the general population in Japan. Neurourol Urodyn. 2009;28:214–8.
14. Berry SH, et al. Prevalence of symptoms of bladder pain syndrome/interstitial cystitis among adult females in the United States. J Urol. 2011;186(2):540–4.
15. Geruso M, Timothy L. Prinz D. Screening in contract design: evidence from the ACA health insurance exchanges. November 10, 2016. SSRN: https://ssrn.com/abstract=2867542 or http://dx.doi.org/10.2139/ssrn.2867542.

Epidemiology Commentary

4

J. Curtis Nickel

In 1990, very little epidemiological data was available to determine the prevalence, much less the incidence of Interstitial Cystitis. The only population based study was from the original author of this chapter, K. J. Oravisto, published in 1975 [1]. In his chapter, Oravisto summarizes some older publications which described small uncontrolled studies including patients with variable and sometimes suspect diagnoses. His landmark 1975 study was not only the first study of its kind but also the only study available to Oravisto at the time he was writing his 1990 chapter. His definition of IC included patients with frequency and pain or discomfort, abnormal biopsy and temporary relief with overdistension of the bladder. In the province of Uusimaa in southern Finland (included city of Helsinki), there were a total of 103 IC patients, 95 women and eight men. The overall prevalence in women (too few men to accurately analyze) over 20 years was 18.6 per 100,000. Over a 10 year period, 64 (61 female) patients were diagnosed with IC; an incidence rate of 1.3 per 100,000 for women over 20 years. He noted that 8% of IC patients in his series were male and when he combined all the series in the literature from 1939 to 1978, the ratio of men to women was noted to be 9.1:1. So how do these figures compare to our contemporary epidemiological studies for this enigmatic condition?

Since 1990, the definition of IC has evolved to now include patients with bladder pain syndrome (initially referred to as Painful Bladder Syndrome) and we have developed validated questionnaires with appropriate inclusion and exclusion criteria to identify, with reasonable accuracy, patients with IC/BPS. But the accuracy of epidemiological studies remains problematic, primarily because the condition is a syndrome (no physical or biochemical marker) and the diagnosis is one of exclusion (excluding confusable diseases that can cause bladder pain and storage symptoms). Since Oravisto's original publication [1] there have been many studies attempting to determine the prevalence and incidence of IC and IC/BPS but they remain difficult to interpret and compare because some are based on unverified self report, others by physician diagnoses (with or without some type of verification) or by identification of BPS symptoms (with or without exclusion of other confusable conditions). There is no wonder then that estimates of prevalence vary widely from 4.5 per 100,000 females in Japan [2], to a questionnaire based study that suggests a figure of 20,000 per 100,000 in US women [3]. Self -report of a previous diagnosis of IC in the 1989 National Household Interview Survey estimated that for women this prevalence figure was 865 per 100,000 [4] while an estimate of IC from the third National Health and Nutrition Examination

J.C. Nickel
Queen's University, Kingston, Canada
e-mail: jcn@queensu.ca

P.M. Hanno et al. (eds.), *Bladder Pain Syndrome – An Evolution*,
https://doi.org/10.1007/978-3-319-61449-6_4

Survey (NHANES III) claimed a remarkably similar estimated prevalence of 850 per 100,000 women [5].

Estimates based on physician diagnoses range from 8 to 197 per 100,000 women [6–8]. Prospective surveys using validated criteria evaluating the prevalence of BPS like symptoms, rather than diagnoses, produce much higher estimates, ranging from 0.8% to 2.7% [9], a range collaborated by other less sensitive older surveys [10]. It is noted, however, that such estimates of IC/BPS prevalence drop drastically if the subjects are examined by urologists to confirm the diagnosis [11, 12]. Using different definitions of IC/BPS also changes the prevalence estimates from 3300 to 11,200 per 100,000 women based on which of three definitions are used [13]. Culture may also play a role, since the estimates vary between the USA (studies described), Europe [14] South Korea [15], China [16] and Japan [2]. The most comprehensive and probably most accurate estimation of the prevalence of BPS symptoms was 2700–6500 per 100,000 based on the sensitivity of the two validated case definitions to identify IC/BPS in 131,691 adult females [17]. Based on the information from epidemiological studies published since Oravisto's chapter in 1990, a reasonable prevalence estimation for patients diagnosed with BPS would be about 100–200 per 100,000 women with a male prevalence of 10–20% of the female estimate. The prevalence of women and men with symptoms suggestive of BPS could be as much as ten to even 100 times more.

Incidence rates for IC/BPs are also difficult to estimate and since Oravisto's estimate of 1.3 per 10,000 women a year, a number of studies have claimed incidence rates ranging from 1.1 to a high of 21 per 100,000 women a year [8, 18, 19].

In conclusion, it appears that IC/BPS is very prevalent, particularly in women. The increased contemporary estimates of prevalence and perhaps incidence compared to that reported by Oravisto in 1990 are most likely related to a less sensitive and restrictive definitions of the syndrome.

References

1. Oravisto KJ. Epidemiology of interstitial cystitis. Ann Chir Gynaecol Fenn. 1975;64(2):75–7.
2. Ito T, Miki M, Yamada T. Interstitial cystitis in Japan. BJU Int. 2000;86(6):634–7.
3. Parsons CL, Tatsis V. Prevalence of interstitial cystitis in young women. Urology. 2004;64(5):866–70.
4. Jones CA, Nyberg L. Epidemiology of interstitial cystitis. Urology. 1997;49(5A Suppl):2–9.
5. Clemens J, Payne C, Pace J. Prevalence of self-reported interstitial cystitis in a nationally representative United States Survey. J Urol. 2005; 173(1):98–102.
6. Bade JJ, Rijcken B, Mensink HJ. Interstitial cystitis in the Netherlands: prevalence, diagnostic criteria and therapeutic preferences. J Urol. 1995;154(6):2035–7.
7. Curhan GC, Speizer FE, Hunter DJ, Curhan SG, Stampfer MJ. Epidemiology of interstitial cystitis: a population based study. J Urol. 1999;161(2):549–52.
8. Clemens JQ, Meenan RT, O'Keeffe Rosetti MC, Brown SO, Gao SY, Calhoun EA. Prevalence of interstitial cystitis symptoms in a managed care population. J Urol. 2005;174(2):576–80.
9. Clemens JQ, Link CL, Eggers PW, Kusek JW, Nyberg LM Jr, McKinlay JB. Prevalence of painful bladder symptoms and effect on quality of life in black, Hispanic and white men and women. J Urol. 2007;177(4):1390–4.
10. Lifford KL, Curhan GC. Prevalence of painful bladder syndrome in older women. Urology. 2009;73(3):494–8.
11. Leppilahti M, Tammela TL, Huhtala H, Auvinen A. Prevalence of symptoms related to interstitial cystitis in women: a population based study in Finland. J Urol. 2002;168(1):139–43.
12. Leppilahti M, Sairanen J, Tammela TL, Aaltomaa S, Lehtoranta K, Auvinen A. Prevalence of clinically confirmed interstitial cystitis in women: a population based study in Finland. J Urol. 2005;174(2):581–3.
13. Clemens J, Meenan R, Rosetti M, Calhoun E. Prevalence and incidence of interstitial cystitis in a managed care population. J Urol. 2005;173:98–102.
14. Temml C, Wehrberger C, Riedl C, Ponholzer A, Marszalek M, Madersbacher S. Prevalence and correlates for interstitial cystitis symptoms in women participating in a health screening project. Eur Urol. 2007;51(3):803–8.
15. Choe JH, Son H, Song YS, Kim JC, Lee JZ, Lee KS. Prevalence of painful bladder syndrome/interstitial cystitis-like symptoms in women: a population-based study in Korea. World J Urol. 2011;29(1):103–8.
16. Song Y, Zhang W, Xu B, Hao L, Song J. Prevalence and correlates of painful bladder syndrome symptoms in Fuzhou Chinese women. Neurourol Urodyn. 2009;28(1):22–5.

17. Berry SH, Elliott MN, Suttorp M, Bogart LM, Stoto MA, Eggers P, et al. Prevalence of symptoms of bladder pain syndrome/interstitial cystitis among adult females in the United States. J Urol. 2011;186(2):540–4.
18. Roberts RO, Bergstralh EJ, Bass SE, Lightner DJ, Lieber MM, Jacobsen SJ. Incidence of physician-diagnosed interstitial cystitis in Olmsted County: a community-based study. BJU Int. 2003;91(3):181–5.
19. Patel R, Calhoun EA, Meenan RT, O'Keeffe Rosetti MC, Kimes T, Clemens JQ. Incidence and clinical characteristics of interstitial cystitis in the community. Int Urogynecol J Pelvic Floor Dysfunct. 2008;19(8):1093–6.

The Prevalence of Bladder Pain Syndrome/Interstitial Cystitis in Italy: The importance of a National Registry

5

Loredana Nasta

Abstract

In the last 30 years, Interstitial Cystitis (IC) diagnostic and etiopathogenetic criteria, as well as its taxonomy, have been strongly debated. Not only internationally, but also within the National Institute of Health (NIH) and especially the National Institute of Diabetes of the Digestive Tract of and Kidney Disease (NIDDK), many changes have occurred.

It is a common opinion that IC epidemiology data are highly inconsistent because of the lack of a shared definition and a valid diagnostic marker.

In 2001, the Italian government recognized this condition as a rare disease, thanks to hard work of Patients' Organization (Associazione Italiana Cistite interstiziale—AICI). The Higher Institute of Health (ISS) was given the task to put in place a National Registry of Rare Diseases (NRRD) as well as the Regional Registries (RR) within the framework of a very complex network consisting of Reference Centers and experts, to collect quality data. The RR are the NRRD infrastructure, an important tool to carry out the network's tracking, the rare diseases surveillance and the data flow analysis where patients receive diagnose and treatments. It will be analyzed the network, NRRD and the data performed in the last 15 years (*Courtesy of ISS*).

5.1 Introduction

Can epidemiology and individual history help us understand the Bladder Pain Syndrome?

This question is important for many people: specialists, scientific societies, Institutions, pharmaceutical companies and patients' associations. The crucial problem of epidemiology is to consider this disease based on the same clinical characteristics and diagnostic criteria. In the last 30 years, diagnostic and etiopathogenetic criteria were highly debated on the international scene. Such criteria have gradually changed over time. New and more complex information, supplemented by results and by "insights" coming from research and clinical practice have been added up.

Thanks to the interest that patients' associations have been raising on this topic in close collaboration with all stakeholders, the debate on chronic pelvic pain of urological origin (UCPPS)

L. Nasta
Italian Interstitial Cystitis Association, Rome, Italy
e-mail: l.nasta@aici-onlus.it

P.M. Hanno et al. (eds.), *Bladder Pain Syndrome – An Evolution*,
https://doi.org/10.1007/978-3-319-61449-6_5

has never stopped in the last three decades. This achievement results from the interest shown by experts and by the most important scientific societies as well as from research funding. It is inevitable to emphasize two important projects called MAPP 1 and MAPP 2 (Multidisciplinary Approach to the Study of Chronic Pelvic Pain Research Network). Their aim is to look into the causes of interstitial cystitis and chronic prostatitis to identify a phenotype. Moreover, it is necessary to explore the theory according to which UCPPS is not necessarily caused by a bladder damage or by the prostate, whereas it might originate from a neurogenic inflammation.

Nonetheless, BPS/IC remains a challenge for the scientific community. There is a lack of consensus on its etiopathogenesis, on diagnostic difficulties, on the lack of diagnostic markers and on the difference among healthcare services in the various countries.

Moreover, in recent years IC taxonomy has changed: initially, it was called Painful Bladder Syndrome (PBS), then Hypersensitive Bladder Syndrome and now BPS.

5.2 Definition from the Nineteenth Century to Date

BPS/IC is a highly complex, strongly disabling, chronic and inflammatory disease. In the past, BPS/IC was considered a rare condition [1]; it is now recognized as the most serious cause of chronic pelvic pain. Two studies carried out by AICI Italy, between 2012 and 2015, together with the Ministry of Social Policy and Welfare, the Catholic University and La Sapienza University of Rome, showed a 10-year diagnostic delay with respect to the onset of symptoms. The same study observed a wide range of recurrent comorbidities and anxious-depressive disorders in 79% of patients. This is an undisputable response to a chronic and complex disease like BPS/IC and its negative impact on the quality of life [2].

Since 1808 to date, much progress has been made. In that year, the disease was described for the first time by Dr. P. S. Physic of Philadelphia. In 1887, the term interstitial cystitis was mentioned for the first time in a paper by Dr. A. J. C. Skene. In 1951, J. P. Bourque proposed to associate the term IC to PBS. This was later accepted by the International Continence Society; again, in 2007 ESSIC and IASP proposed a radical replacement with the term BPS.

The inclusion and exclusion diagnostic criteria, established by NIDDK in 1987, followed more or less the same destiny. Subject to constant criticism for almost 10 years, because they were considered too stringent, they have remained the diagnostic foundation in the context of research until 2003, despite the progress made in those years. Two papers published in 1999 showed that the criteria established by NIDDK-NIH were missing about two thirds of BPS/IC cases. Sixty percent of patients, despite a BPS/IC diagnosis made by clinical experts, were not included in NIDDK research criteria. Moreover, children and adolescents under the age of 18 were not included at all [3]. In 2001, a thought-provoking article was published. Its authors wondered whether time had come to review diagnostic criteria and, therefore, the IC definition [4].

5.3 Epidemiology

As previously mentioned, BPS/IC epidemiology studies suffered from several problems in the course of the past decades. This caused problems in the interpretation of the scientific literature. Pelvic pain of bladder origin can be similar to other diseases or causes (post-surgery, trauma, sexual abuse, endometriosis, vulvodinia, abacterial prostatitis, prostatodinia, confusable diseases). The terminology used for PBS actually includes symptoms related to many painful urological conditions, including IC. Research methods also vary. They are undoubtedly influenced by inadequate criteria lacking a universal acceptance. This is the reason why studies on the incidence and prevalence of BPS/IC are so inconsistent.

Oravisto, for example, uses emptying and histological criteria; Held and Bade use the same method, i.e. they send questionnaires by mail and review clinical records; Jones uses clinical records only; Curhan and Ito use questionnaires sent by mail, other authors make use of interviews. The first epidemiology study conducted in Finland in 1975, was certainly the most important one because it covered a population of about one million. The prevalence of the disease among women turned out to be 1.81 every 10,000 inhabitants, whereas the prevalence in both sexes was equal to 1.06 cases per 10,000 [5]. Jones and Nyberg [6], in a comparison of three epidemiology studies, show that different criteria had been employed to define an IC case and no study had employed NIH research criteria. The result is a considerable variability of prevalence rates. For example, in Finland, they used only clinical records (1 case every 10,000 inhabitants); the United States sent a questionnaire by mail (3 every 10,000); the NIH used a self-completed questionnaire (51 every 10,000) and so did other countries in the rest of the world [7]. In the Netherlands, IC prevalence is determined through a questionnaire completed by urologists. Prevalence varies from 0.8 to 1.6/10,000 women patients. This finding is in line with European data but lower if compared to the United States [8].

In 2005, Kusek et al. [9] complained about the small number of epidemiology studies due to an uncommon clinical condition and to the long time elapsing between the onset of symptoms and diagnosis.

Another early study in the United States demonstrated the potential extension of what was considered a rare disease [1]. The authors of this study, dating back to 1987, concluded that there were 43,500 to 90,000 undiagnosed IC cases in the USA, exactly twice as much as in Finland. Finally, Japan reported a prevalence of 0.12/10,000 inhabitants, even lower than in Europe and in the United States [10]. This finding was endorsed by a further study conducted by a group of researchers in South Korea [11].

In other words, prevalence varies from a minimum of 1.8: 10,000 inhabitants up to an estimated 45–51 cases every 10,000 inhabitants [12]. These estimates, rather than representing very significant differences in terms of prevalence, should make us reflect on the various methods used to define an IC case and their limited reliability. Most study end with hypothetical estimates. This presupposes that millions of patients suffering from BPS/IC are still in search of a diagnosis. However, a continuous awareness-raising effort by patients' associations among primary care physicians, specialists and on the media, the advent of the Internet, social networks and disease-specific blogs, have played an important role in achieving an increasingly early diagnosis.

5.4 Establishing the Network and the National Registry

In 2000, the European Parliament and the Council of the European Union defined Rare Diseases (RD) as conditions with a low prevalence threshold (50/100,000 inhabitants in the EC) and a high degree of complexity [13], differently from the rates reported by United States (7.5/10,000) and Japan (4/10,000). In May 2001, the Italian Ministry of Health approved Ministerial Decree 279. Italy became the first country in Europe and worldwide to officially establish a very complex national network. Reference centers for individual diseases were identified and a National Registry of Rare Diseases (NRRD) was established. This latter had the objective of collecting data on the prevalence, incidence and risk factors of the various diseases listed by the Decree. BPS/IC was included under code RJ0030 and received the Orphanet code ORPHA37202.

But how is the network organized? As a first step, the NRRD was entrusted to the Higher Institute of Health to collect epidemiology data (first of all, the number of cases of a rare disease and their distribution nationwide). This helps define the size of the problem, estimate the delay in the time to diagnosis and the healthcare migration pattern by patients. The average diagnostic delay of a RD may in fact be quite long, with an average estimated time of around 5 years after the onset of the first symptoms. Shortening this delay means to significantly improve the quality of life of patients and establish more reliable and effective care and therapeutich paths. A late diagnosis can be explained by possible etiological factors, as well as by the incidence and/or prevalence of the disease itself [14]. The second step was the identification of BPS/IC centers of reference, the only ones authorized to certify the diagnosis and administer therapies. These centers had to meet stringent criteria, including a proven previous 10 year knowledge of the disease. The third step was the development of diagnostic and care therapeutic protocols. These had to be agreed upon by the centers and by the Patients' Associations. The Ministry of Health funded a 15 million project specifically focused on BPS/IC. In 2007, the Presidency of the Council of Ministers promoted the establishment of such Registries in the 20 Italian regions.

The accredited centers began entering patient data in the regional registries (RR). RRs periodically send data to NRRD.

5.5 How the Registry Works

The establishment of a BPS/IC multicenter registry can provide important "insights" on the prevalence and characteristics of patients to allow a rigorous assessment of their response to interventions. Furthermore, NRRD is a fundamental tool to study the epidemiology of BPS/IC, as well as to promote a debate among specialists, evalute the effectiveness and costs of any planned public health initiative. A strong motivation to enter data and keep the Center qualification was the proven existence of a large flow of patients. Patients, on their turn, can receive healthcare and therapy for free only if they are part of the registry. NRRD, to improve the network performance, put at the disposal of Centers and Regions a data collection computerized system for free. This latter uses a common language, through a software developed on a user-friendly web platform. It is fully compliant with security and confidentiality standards for the treatment of sensitive data. Data are collected through an online form. Data are then sent to NRRD and access is authorized by a password. The minimum data set provides for mandatory fields, both for demographics and for the pathology features. An important requirement of the operating system used by NRRD is the exchange of information with other flows of farmacosurveillance and other disease registries, in view of a European comparative analysis.

NRRD activities are included in the National Statistical Plan. This is extraordinarily important in so far as it represents a commitment by the System to produce official, high quality statistical information.

5.6 Prevalence

We report Registry data for 2014 and 2015 in five significant regions—Lombardy, Piedmont, Tuscany, Marche and Lazio—as well as the overall NRRD data reported for 2013–2014. NRRD results for 2015–2016 are still under evaluation.

The first sample regards Lombardy RR: in 2014, the registry counted 345 patients affected by BPS/IC, 25 males, 316 females and 4 deceased patients, with a prevalence of 0.27 males out of 100,000 and a prevalence of 3.49 females out of 100,000. The total prevalence was 3.77 out of 100,000 [15]. In 2015, the registry counted 386 patients—25 males, 355 females and 6 deceased patients. The prevalence was equal to 0.24/100,000 for males and 3.54/100,000 for females. The total prevalence appeared to be equal to 3.79 out of 100,000 [16].

In 2015, the Piedmont RR counted 116 patients, with a prevalence of 2.63 out of 100,000.

In 2015, the Tuscany RR consisted of 91 patients with a BPS/IC diagnosis out of a population of 3,744,398. The prevalence was equal to 2.43/100,000.

In 2015, the Marche RR registered 77 patients with a prevalence of 4, 98 out of 100,000.

In 2014, the Lazio RR registered 289 BPS/IC patients, equal to only 1.7% of all RD diagnosed [17]. In 2015, the number of patients suffering from BPS/IC rose to 305 but the percentage dropped to 1.6% [18] with a prevalence of 5.1/100,000.

In 2013–2014, NRRD had 1192 patients in a population of almost 61 million. The Italian Prevalence results 1.9 out of 100,000.

Table 5.1 Prevalence of BPS/IC in different regions and nationwide in Italy

Data between 2014 and 2015	Number of patients in the Registry	Number of inhabitants according to ISTAT	Prevalence every 10,000
Lombardy Region Registry, 2014	341 patients	9,032,554 inhabitants	3.7/100,000
Lombardy Region Registry, 2015	380 patients	10,008,349 inhabitants	3.8/100,000
Piedmont Region Registry, 2015	116 patients	4,404,246 inhabitants	2.6/100,000
Tuscany Region Registry, 2015	91 patients	3,744,398 inhabitants	2.4/100,000
Marche Region Registry, 2015	77 patients	1,543,752 inhabitants	5/100,000
Lazio Region Registry, 2014	289 patients	5,892,425 inhabitants	4.9/100,000
Lazio Region Registry, 2015	305 patients	5,888,472 inhabitants	5.1/100,000
National Registry, 2013–2014	1192 patients	60,795,612 inhabitants	1.9/100,000
National Registry, 2015–2016	Data collected under evaluation	Data collected under evaluation	

In 2015–2016, NRRD data have been collected and they are under evaluation (Table 5.1).

Conclusions

In spite of a certain degree of statistical error, these results indicate that BPS/IC is not a common occurrence in the Italian population. It is widely agreed that a disease registry is a valuable source of information both for epidemiology and for public health. Moreover, it helps estimate the diagnostic delay, one of the key research areas related to this type of diseases. In the next 2 years, it will be interesting to evaluate the prevalence pattern of BPS/IC in Italy, in view of a comparison between Italian data and other European registries.

References

1. Forrest JB. Epidemiology and quality of life. J Reprod Med. 2006;51(3 Suppl):227–33.
2. Nasta L, Montagnoli S, Avolio M. Chapter 29: Exploratory Research on the social costs and care for patients with bladder pain syndrome/interstitial cystitis. In: Nordling J, Wyndaele JJ, van de Merwe JP, et al., editors. BPS: a guide for clinicians; 2013.
3. Hanno PM, Landis JR, Matthews-Cook Y, et al. The diagnosis of interstitial cystitis revisited: lessons learned from the National Institutes of Health Interstitial Cystitis Database study. J Urol. 1999;161(2):553–7.
4. Agarwal M, O'Reilly PH, Dixon RA. Interstitial cystitis—a time for revision of name and diagnostic criteria in the new millennium? BJU Int. 2001;88(4):348–50.
5. Held PJ, Hanno PM, Wein AJ. Epidemiology of interstitial cystitis (2). Chapter 4. Springer; 1990.
6. Jones CA, Nyberg L. Epidemiology of interstitial cystitis. Urology. 1997;49(5A Suppl):2–9.
7. Oravisto KJ. Epidemiology of interstitial cystitis. Ann Chir Gynaecol Fenn. 1975;64(2):75–7.
8. Bade JJ, Rijcken B, Mensink HJ. Interstitial cystitis in the Netherlands: prevalence, diagnostic criteria and therapeutic preferences. J Urol. 1995;154(6):2035–7, discussion 2037–8.
9. Kusek JW, Nyberg LM. The epidemiology of interstitial cystitis: is it time to expand our definition? Urology. 2001;57(6 Suppl 1):95–9.
10. Ito T, Miki M, Yamada T. Interstitial cystitis in Japan. BJU Int. 2000;86(6):634–7.
11. Choe JH, Son H, Song YS, et al. Prevalence of painful bladder syndrome/interstitial cystitis-like symptoms in women: a population-based study in Korea. World J Urol. 2011;29(1):103–8.
12. Curhan GC, Speizer FE, Hunter DJ, et al. Epidemiology of interstitial cystitis: a population based study. J Urol. 1999;161(2):549–52.
13. RE 141/00-http://eur-lex.europa.eu/legal-content/IT/ALL/?uri=CELEX:32000R0141
14. http://www.iss.it/binary/cnmr4/cont/ISTISAN_RNMR_2011.pdf

15. http://malattierare.marionegri.it/images/RRMR_ESENZIONI/2014_12_31_relmar.pdf
16. http://malattierare.marionegri.it/images/RRMR_ESENZIONI/2015_12_31_relmar.pdf
17. http://www.regione.lazio.it/malattierare/allegati/rapporto_lazio_malattie_rare_2014.pdf
18. http://www.regione.lazio.it/malattierare/allegati/rapporto_lazio_malattie_rare_2015.pdf

Interstitial Cystitis: Animal Models

6

Tony Buffington, Michael R. Ruggieri, and David J. Klumpp

In 1990, although the etiology and pathogenesis of the condition then referred to as "interstitial cystitis" (IC) was admitted to be largely or even completely unknown, the widely held implicit working assumptions held that it is a bladder disease. These assumptions implied that if we could discover and correct what was wrong with the bladder itself then we could cure the condition. These assumptions have proved to be largely off base. At that time, the previous suggestions that IC might have a primarily autoimmune or infectious etiology were largely abandoned. The autoimmune hypothesis still remains but has yet to be either been proven nor disproven conclusively.

Application of highly refined and exquisitely sensitive molecular techniques have essentially disproved the possibility of an infectious etiology. Because IC was assumed to be a bladder disease, investigations turned to "the relationship between IC and the properties of the surface of the bladder lumen." Considerable evidence existed that the quality of the bladder surface mucin protects the bladder from bacterial colonization and from the irritative effects of noxious substances (e.g., H^+, K^+) in urine, so studies of mucin removal were conducted in healthy rabbits. In response to anecdotal reports that the antibiotic nitrofurantoin, commonly used to treat urinary tract infections, may act as a surface-active agent disrupting the bladder surface mucin and inducing IC, investigations attempted to use chronic nitrofurantoin administration to create an animal model of IC by studying both the acute and chronic effect of nitrofurantoin on the urinary bladder of rabbits. No such disruptive effect of nitrofurantoin on the bladder surface mucin was found. These investigations concluded that although experimental pathologies such as 1 h of bladder ischemia or overdistension and 1 week of partial bladder outlet obstruction, caused significant decreases in anti-adherence characteristics of the bladder mucosa, "whether these perturbations are transient or not remains the subject of further investigation." The chapter concluded by proposing that the use of animal models to study isolated symptoms of IC would assist and greatly speed the process of investigation.

T. Buffington, DVM, PhD, DACVN (emeritus) (✉)
Clinical Professor, Department of Medicine and Epidemiology, UC Davis School of Veterinary Medicine, Davis, CA, USA

Emeritus Professor of Veterinary Clinical Sciences, The Ohio State University, Columbus, OH, USA
e-mail: drbuffington@ucdavis.edu

M.R. Ruggieri, Sr., PhD
Associate Professor, Department of Anatomy and Cell Biology, Lewis Katz School of Medicine, Temple University, Philadelphia, PA, USA

D.J. Klumpp, PhD
Associate Professor of Urology and Microbiology-Immunology, Feinberg School of Medicine, Northwestern University, Chicago, IL, USA

P.M. Hanno et al. (eds.), *Bladder Pain Syndrome – An Evolution*,
https://doi.org/10.1007/978-3-319-61449-6_6

6.1 What Did We Get Right?

The authors of the chapter rightly summarized the work at the time of publication of the book, and presciently recognized that no one animal model of IC was likely to recapitulate all of the findings present in patients with the syndrome. Indeed, expectation that any animal model of a condition of unknown etiology and obscure pathogenesis can recapitulate all aspects of the clinical condition is a gross over expectation. The best that can be expected is to be able to create animal models with known etiologic and pathogenic mechanisms for specific symptoms of the condition and then to test whether these same mechanisms are involved in clinical cases.

The possibility was raised that "agents in the urine peculiar to patients with IC may initiate the pathogenic process." Repeated infusion of urine from IC patients into the normal rabbit bladder has since been found to induce the classic cystoscopic appearance of interstitial cystitis [1, 2] and a number of abnormalities in the urine and urothelial cell structure and function have since been reported (see [3] for review).

6.2 Where Were We Off Base?

The mucin and glycosaminoglycan hypotheses ultimately were not supported [4–6]. Although bladder injuries certainly can be induced in animals, it remains mostly unknown if the resulting abnormalities represent models of cause, coincidence, or consequence of IC, limiting their relevance to IC in humans. That said, the recent reports of post-UTI chronic pain demonstrate that certain strains of E. coli have the capacity to induce pelvic pain behavior in mice that persists long after bacterial clearance, consistent with the prevalence of UTI history in IC patients [7]. Additionally, neonatal bladder inflammation can result in long-term visceral pain and altered responses of spinal neurons in adult rats [8, 9].

Two different strategies have been deployed to investigate IC in animals in the intervening years. One approach largely followed the recommendations of Chap. 14; the other was to investigate a (potentially) naturally occurring model of IC in domestic cats that was called "Feline Urologic Syndrome".

In addition to continued studies of induced bladder injury, studies of the role(s) of environmental factors on the development of IC also have appeared. For example, increased voiding frequency was reported in corticotrophin releasing factor overexpressing mice [10], and both water avoidance stress [11, 12], and adverse early life experiences [13] have been found to result in irritative voiding signs in rodents.

Studies of the naturally occurring model of IC began with the same goal. Cats with sufficiently severe disease that their owners had elected euthanasia were obtained as donations, and then transported and housed in the vivarium of The Ohio State University and studied [14]. Three important initial observations were that many of the cats had variable combinations of signs of comorbid disorders (as is the case with humans with the syndrome), that these signs routinely resolved with housing in the enriched environment of the vivarium, and that they recurred in response to disruptions in the cats' surroundings [15]. These findings resulted in the hypothesis that these cats, rather than having a bladder disease, might have a disease of the central nervous system that was afflicting the bladder and various other body systems (similar hypotheses have been investigated in humans [8, 14, 16]). We tested this hypothesis in a prospective observational study of "multimodal environmental modification" (MEMO) in client owned cats with the syndrome, and found that it led to significant reductions in signs referable to the bladder, as well as to other affected organs [17]. The MEMO approach subsequently has become the standard of care for cats with IC in veterinary medicine [18].

Like the induced bladder injury models, IC in cats also has limitations as a model of IC in humans. One is the seemingly different gender distribution between affected males and females of the two species. In cats, both genders are affected roughly equally, whereas early studies in humans suggested that 90% of patients were women [19]. Recent reports, however, suggest that the sex difference in humans may not be as large as originally thought [19, 20], if it exists at all [21, 22]. Additionally, affected cats are not easy to acquire without both veterinarian and owner cooperation, are more expensive to maintain in laboratory animal facilities than are rodents, are outbred, and lack many of the molecular tools available for rodents. Despite these limitations, studies of cats with IC have duplicated many results obtained in humans with IC, and even predicted some abnormalities that were subsequently found in humans with the syndrome [23, 24], in ways not currently possible in humans or induced animal models [25].

6.3 What Seminal Publications Changed Our Thinking?

This publication [26] led to investigations of the roles of the HPA axis in cats with IC. Consideration of the role of adverse early life experiences in IC and related disorders as spurred by these publications [8, 9, 27]. This publication [28] led to consideration of the role of epigenetic modulation of gene expression in central sensitization. Development of the MEMO approach was helped by this publication [29].

6.4 Where Do We Go from Here?

Based on studies of IC in cats, a human "version" of the MEMO approach developed to treat cats was tested in humans with fibromyalgia (FM), [30] a disorder commonly comorbid with IC [31]. Nine patients with FM were provided with individual and group health and wellness coaching (HWC) telephonically for 12 months. We used the Revised Fibromyalgia Impact Questionnaire (FIQR) to measure health and quality of life, and the Brief Pain Inventory-Short Form (BPI) to measure pain intensity and interference with function. We also documented total and rheumatology-related health encounters using electronic medical records. All nine patients finished the HWC protocol, and their FIQR scores improved by 35% ($P = 0.001$), and BPI scores decreased by 31% for severity ($P = 0.02$), and 44% for interference ($P = 0.006$). Importantly, health care utilization declined by 86% ($P = 0.006$) for total and 78% ($P < 0.0001$) for rheumatology-related encounters, suggesting that the HWC program added to standard FM therapy produced clinically significant improvements in all measures. Such improvements do not typically occur spontaneously in FM patients, suggesting that HWC deserves further consideration as an intervention for FM, and for patients with IC as well.

References

1. Kohn IJ, Filer-Maerten S, Whitmore KE, Hanno PM, Ruggieri MR. Lack of effect following repeated in vivo exposure of the rabbit urinary bladder to urine from interstitial cystitis patients at low infusion volumes. Neurourol Urodyn. 1998;17(2):147–52.
2. Ruggieri MR, Chelsky MJ, Rosen SI, Shickley TJ, Hanno PM. Current findings and future research avenues in the study of interstitial cystitis. Urol Clin North Am. 1994;21(1):163–76.
3. Keay SK, Birder LA, Chai TC. Evidence for bladder urothelial pathophysiology in functional bladder disorders. Biomed Res Int. 2014;2014:865463.
4. Chew DJ, Bartges JW, Adams LG, Kruger JM, Buffington CAT. Evaluation of pentosan polysulfate sodium for Feline Interstitial Cystitis: a randomized, placebo-controlled clinical trial. In preparation. 2008.
5. Nickel JC, Herschorn S, Whitmore KE, Forrest JB, Hu P, Friedman AJ, et al. Pentosan polysulfate sodium for treatment of interstitial cystitis/bladder pain syndrome: insights from a randomized, double-blind, placebo-controlled study. J Urol. 2014;193(3):857–62.
6. Hanno PM, Wolf S. Guidelines Q&A: diagnosis and treatment of interstitial cystitis/bladder pain syndrome. Health Policy Brief. 2014;21(1).
7. Rudick CN, Jiang M, Yaggie RE, Pavlov VI, Done J, Heckman CJ, et al. O-antigen modulates infection-induced pain states. PLoS One. 2012;7(8):e41273.
8. DeBerry J, Ness TJ, Robbins MT, Randich A. Inflammation-induced enhancement of the visceromotor reflex to urinary bladder distention: modulation by endogenous opioids and the effects of early-in-life experience with bladder inflammation. J Pain. 2007;8(12):914–23.
9. Randich A, Uzzell T, DeBerry JJ, Ness TJ. Neonatal urinary bladder inflammation produces adult bladder hypersensitivity. J Pain. 2006;7(7):469–79.
10. Million M, Wang L, Stenzel-Poore MP, Coste S, Yuan PQ, Lamy C, et al. Enhanced pelvic responses to stressors in female CRF-overexpressing mice. Am J Physiol Regul Integr Comp Physiol. 2007;292(4):R1429–38.

11. Larauche M, Mulak A, Tache Y. Stress and visceral pain: from animal models to clinical therapies. Exp Neurol. 2012;233(1):49–67.
12. Lee UJ, Ackerman AL, Wu A, Zhang R, Leung J, Bradesi S, et al. Chronic psychological stress in high-anxiety rats induces sustained bladder hyperalgesia. Physiol Behav. 2015;139:541–8.
13. Pierce AN, Di Silvestro ER, Eller OC, Wang R, Ryals JM, Christianson JA. Urinary bladder hypersensitivity and dysfunction in female mice following early life and adult stress. Brain Res. 1639;2016:58–73.
14. Buffington CA. Idiopathic cystitis in domestic cats-beyond the lower urinary tract. J Vet Intern Med. 2011;25(4):784–96.
15. Stella JL, Lord LK, Buffington CA. Sickness behaviors in response to unusual external events in healthy cats and cats with feline interstitial cystitis. J Am Vet Med Assoc. 2011;238(1):67–73.
16. Warren JW, Howard FM, Cross RK, Good JL, Weissman MM, Wesselmann U, et al. Antecedent nonbladder syndromes in case-control study of interstitial cystitis/painful bladder syndrome. Urology. 2009;73(1):52–7.
17. Buffington CAT, Westropp JL, Chew DJ, Bolus RR. Clinical evaluation of multimodal environmental modification in the management of cats with lower urinary tract signs. J Feline Med Surg. 2006;8:261–8.
18. Carney HC, Sadek TP, Curtis TM, Halls V, Heath S, Hutchison P, et al. AAFP and ISFM guidelines for diagnosing and solving house-soiling behavior in cats. J Feline Med Surg. 2014;16(7):579–98.
19. Jones CA, Nyberg L. Epidemiology of interstitial cystitis. Urology. 1997;49(5A):2–9.
20. Clemens JQ, Meenan RT, Rosetti MC, Gao SY, Calhoun EA. Prevalence and incidence of interstitial cystitis in a managed care population. J Urol. 2005;173(1):98–102; discussion.
21. Miller JL, Rothman I, Bavendam TG, Berger RE. Prostatodynia and interstitial cystitis: one and the same? Urology. 1994;45:587–90.
22. Suskind AM, Berry SH, Ewing BA, Elliott MN, Suttorp MJ, Clemens JQ. The prevalence and overlap of interstitial cystitis/bladder pain syndrome and chronic prostatitis/chronic pelvic pain syndrome in men: results of the RAND Interstitial Cystitis Epidemiology male study. J Urol. 2013;189(1):141–5.
23. Dimitrakov J, Joffe HV, Soldin SJ, Bolus R, Buffington CA, Nickel JC. Adrenocortical hormone abnormalities in men with chronic prostatitis/chronic pelvic pain syndrome. Urology. 2008;71(2):261–6.
24. Twiss C, Kilpatrick L, Craske M, Buffington CA, Ornitz E, Rodriguez LV, et al. Increased startle responses in interstitial cystitis: evidence for central hyperresponsiveness to visceral related threat. J Urol. 2009;181(5):2127–33.
25. Buffington CAT. From animal data to human practice. In: Messelink B, Baranowski A, Hughes J, editors. Abdominal and pelvic pain: from definition to best practice. Washington, DC: IASP Press; 2014. p. 23–35.
26. Heim C, Ehlert U, Hellhammer DH. The potential role of hypocortisolism in the pathophysiology of stress-related bodily disorders. Psychoneuroendocrinology. 2000;25(1):1–35.
27. Gluckman PD, Hanson MA. Mismatch: why our world no longer fits our bodies. Oxford: Oxford University Press; 2006. p. 304.
28. Weaver ICG, Cervoni N, Champagne FA, D'Alessio AC, Sharma S, Seckl JR, et al. Epigenetic programming by maternal behavior. Nat Neurosci. 2004;7(8):847–54.
29. Koolhaas JM, Korte SM, De Boer SF, Van Der Vegt BJ, Van Reenen CG, Hopster H, et al. Coping styles in animals: current status in behavior and stress-physiology. Neurosci Biobehav Rev. 1999;23(7):925–35.
30. Hackshaw KV, Plans-Pujolras M, Rodriguez-Saona LE, Moore MA, Jackson EK, Sforzo GA, et al. A pilot study of health and wellness coaching for fibromyalgia. BMC Musculoskelet Disord. 2016;17(1):457.
31. Clauw DJ, Schmidt M, Radulovic D, Singer A, Katz P, Bresette J. The relationship between fibromyalgia and interstitial cystitis. J Psychiatr Res. 1997;31(1):125–31.

Etiology: Etiological and Pathogenic Theories of Interstitial Cystitis/Bladder Pain Syndrome

7

Jørgen Nordling, David Staskin, and Naoki Yoshimura

When this chapter was first written in 1990, Interstitial Cystitis (IC) had no established universally accepted definition and no widely agreed upon diagnostic criteria. Consequently, patients receiving the clinical diagnosis constituted a wide range of different phenotypes of urinary frequency, urgency or pain—a diagnosis established primarily based on symptoms—depending on the diagnostic criteria created by the individual doctor making the diagnosis.

The lack of established sensitive or specific objective symptoms or signs is evident in the NIDDK criteria published in this book in 1990. The NIDDK criteria were primarily established for selecting patients for scientific studies. Because of the desire to not exclude any subjects with predominant urgency "or" pain from potential treatment—these criteria permitted the investigator with subjects to include a wide range of the symptom spectrum—but did not provide the clinician with a specific criterion for the diagnosis of patients.

In the NIDDK criteria **PAIN** or **URGENCY** were the two symptoms selected to be necessary for inclusion into clinical studies of IC. Important was the word "**or**", indicating that patients with the symptom of urgency, but no pain were eligible to receive the diagnosis. Taking a retrospective look at the last 30 years, this definition permitted many to be diagnosed as having IC, who since the introduction of Overactive Bladder Syndrome (OAB) in 2002 [1] would be diagnosed as having idiopathic OAB. Today this is still the case in many countries in Asia, where the NIDDK criteria until very recently were the diagnostic criteria for IC [2].

This is only one example of the heterogeneity of IC patient populations of that time. The desire for broad inclusion criteria while establishing the etiology of the disease made the establishment of diagnostic criteria and therapeutic responses highly challenging and almost with certainty doomed to be a failure. Chapter 6 which provided many etiologic theories and no positive conclusions confirms this dilemma.

ESSIC introduced in 2008 Bladder Pain Syndrome (BPS) instead of IC [3] including a definition of the disease and a classification system. Due to problems with regulatory authorities, reimbursement, etc., the terminology utilized today is often BPS/IC or IC/BPS employing the ESSIC definition or another modification of this without changing the traditional definition. Nevertheless, BPS is still a heterogeneous patient group and the search for one or more unifying etiologies has still not been very successful.

7.1 What Did We Get Right?

In the original chapter the term used was "Painful Bladder disease including interstitial cystitis" and attention was thereby brought to the problem

J. Nordling (✉) • D. Staskin • N. Yoshimura
Department of Urology, Herlev Hospital,
Herlev, Denmark
e-mail: jnordling@dadlnet.dk

P.M. Hanno et al. (eds.), *Bladder Pain Syndrome – An Evolution*,
https://doi.org/10.1007/978-3-319-61449-6_7

of definition and delineation of the disease. Nevertheless, studies on etiology were on diverse patient populations, and therefore all negative.

The theoretical etiologies proposed in the1990 edition:

Infection
Extra vesical foci or infection
Allergic, immune or autoimmune disorders
Defective cytoprotection
Toxic agents in the urine
Genetic deviancies
Endocrinological disturbances
Lymphatic obstruction
Vascular obstruction
Neurogenic disturbances
Psychiatric disease

The etiologies under discussion in 2016 are more or less the same (ICI 2016 Tokyo):

Immune cell activation
Increased permeability of the urothelium due to urothelial dysfunction/GAG layer defects
Inhibition of Bladder Urothelial Cell Proliferation
Infection
Neurobiology/Pelvic Crosstalk
Urinary Toxic Agents
Hypoxia
Genetics

The only proposed etiologies in 1990 not still in consideration are: Endocrinological disturbances and psychiatric disease.

It is comforting, that at least psychiatric disease is out of the list today.

7.2 Where Were We Off Base?

1. Overactive Bladder Syndrome and other Lower Urinary Tract Symptoms: The inclusion of a large variety of lower urinary tract disorders—comprised of the symptoms of urgency, frequency, nocturia, without pain. The inclusion of patients with frequency and urgency and without pain broadened inclusion criteria and increased the heterogeneity of the population.
2. Abnormal cystoscopy including the findings of "glomerulation" and "Hunner's Ulcer": This subgroup originally defined by the specific findings of submucosal hemorrhage or Hunner's Lesions in the bladder was not given the status of a recognized sub-group, but were considered more severe forms of the disease on a spectrum. This assumption made the search for a common etiology for the disorder rather meaningless. No doubt, we may have been far more advanced in our understanding of the Hunner Lesion group, if patients with Hunner Lesion had been studied as a distinct disease [4].

   It is today believed, that the etiology of BPS is more complex than believed in 1990 [5–8].
3. Urodynamic findings: Although the presence of urinary frequency implies decreased voiding volume and therefore decreased bladder capacity there was no specific criteria concerning the "sensory" component of the disease process. Even in 2016 the criteria to differentiate patients with afferent neurological disorders emanating from the mucosa, submucosa or muscle—or a group with submucosal fibrosis and changes in bladder compliance has not been established. Bladder capacity by voided volumes is not required. Cystometry under anesthesia with or without pharmacological provocation has not been studied.

7.3 What Seminal Publications Changed Our Thinking?

The paper from Magnus Fall in 1987 [9] did not attract much attention at that time, but read today it really underlines the importance of phenotyping in syndromes like BPS in order to make progress in the study of a probably very heterogeneous patient group.

7.4 Where Do We Go from Here?

Hunner Lesion patients must in the future be studied separately as a distinct disease. Because a huge proportion of patients with BPS without Hunner Lesion also have other pain syndromes the tendency today is to look on this patient group as having a more generalized somatic disorder and should therefore be evaluated as such. The Multidisciplinary Approach to Pelvic Pain (MAPP) study by NIDDK (https://www.niddk.nih.gov/news/research-updates/Pages/multi%E2%80%91disciplinary-approach-study-chronic-pelvic-pain.aspx) is such a study, which might bring some more light into this area.

References

1. Abrams P, Cardozo L, Fall M, Griffiths D, Rosier P, Ulmsten U, van Kerrebroeck P, Victor A, Wein A. The standardization of terminology of lower urinary tract function. Neurourol Urodyn. 2002;21(2):167–78.
2. Homma Y, Ueda T, Ito T, Takei M, Tomoe H. Japanese guideline for diagnosis and treatment of interstitial cystitis. Int J Urol. 2009;16(1):4–16.
3. van de Merwe JP, Nordling J, Bouchelouche P, Bouchelouche K, Cervigni M, Daha LK, et al. Diagnostic criteria, classification, and nomenclature for painful bladder syndrome/interstitial cystitis: an ESSIC proposal. Eur Urol. 2008;53(1):60–7.
4. Fall M, Logadottir Y, Peeker R. Interstitial cystitis is bladder pain syndrome with Hunner's lesion. Int J Urol. 2014;21(Suppl 1):79–82.
5. Alagiri M, Chottiner S, Ratner V, Slade D, Hanno PM. Interstitial cystitis: unexplained associations with other chronic disease and pain syndromes. Urology. 1997;49(5A Suppl):52–7.
6. Aaron LA, Buchwald D. A review of the evidence for overlap among unexplained clinical conditions. Ann Intern Med. 2001;134(9 Pt 2):868–81.
7. Clauw DJ. The pathogenesis of chronic pain and fatigue syndromes, with special reference to fibromyalgia. Med Hypotheses. 1995;44(5):369–78.
8. Sand PK. Proposed pathogenesis of painful bladder syndrome/interstitial cystitis. J Reprod Med. 2006;51(3 Suppl):234–40.
9. Fall M, Johansson SL, Aldenborg F. Chronic interstitial cystitis: a heterogeneous syndrome. J Urol. 1987;137(1):35–8.

7.4 Where Do We Go from Here?

References

8 Differences in Clinical Features and Histopathology in BPS/IC with and without Hunner Lesions

Christina Kåbjörn-Gustafsson and Ralph Peeker

8.1 Bladder Pain Syndrome With or Without Hunner Lesions

The understanding of interstitial cystitis (IC) has changed a lot since the term was first introduced by Skene as early as in 1887 [1]. Guy L. Hunner described a symptom complex of bladder pain associated with an elusive cystoscopic feature, the Hunner ulcer, almost exactly 100 years ago [2]. A couple of decades later things became a lot more confusing when John Hand presented a large series of IC patients noticing that IC did not comprise just one single entity [3]. Some 40 years ago Messing and Stamey believed that there might be an early form of the disease, displaying the so-called submucosal glomerulations, potentially progressing into the well-known classic disease [4]. This notion has subsequently been considered unrealistic since progression from the so-called 'early form' to the classic ulcerous form or end stage disease (bladder contracture) actually never has been reported. Conversely, during the recent decades it has become increasingly clear that the different forms of IC indeed represent completely different pathological entities, despite sharing similar symptomatology and the same chronic course [5–8]. In a recent report, Killinger et al. failed to reveal any significant differences in pain patterns between the two subtypes [9].The differences between the two subtypes are reflected in clinical manifestation and age distribution [7, 8]. It has also been reported that the two subtypes respond differently to many treatment procedures [8]. Koziol et al. supported the contention of heterogeneity of interstitial cystitis by observations based on epidemiological data relating to demographics, risk factors, symptoms, pain and psychosocial factors [6], and, more recently, Peters et al. demonstrated notable differences between the two subtypes in the number of comorbid diagnoses as well as symptoms [10]. In these reports, subjects with Hunner disease were significantly older.

The percentage of classic and nonulcer disease, respectively, of the total number of patients with interstitial cystitis is under debate. Messing and Stamey reported classic interstitial cystitis to account for about half of all patients with interstitial cystitis [4]. Later, the Hunner type has been considered a rare finding, accounting for 5–10% of cases of interstitial cystitis [11]. However, Koziol et al. presented a very large series in

C. Kåbjörn-Gustafsson, M.D., Ph.D. (✉)
Institute of Biomedicine, Gothenburg University, Solkullevägen 10, SE 43833 Landvetter, Sweden
e-mail: christina.kabjorngustafsson@gmail.com

R. Peeker
Department of Urology, Institute of Clinical Sciences, Sahlgrenska Academy at the University of Gothenburg, SE 41345 Göteborg, Sweden

P.M. Hanno et al. (eds.), *Bladder Pain Syndrome – An Evolution*,
https://doi.org/10.1007/978-3-319-61449-6_8

which classic interstitial cystitis accounted for approximately 20% [6].

Endoscopically, classic IC displays reddened mucosal areas often associated with small vessels radiating towards a central scar which ruptures with increasing bladder distension. Nonulcer IC, on the other hand, displays a normal bladder mucosa at initial cystoscopy. The development of glomerulations after hydrodistension is considered to be a positive diagnostic sign. However, a report by Waxman showed that there was no difference in cystoscopic appearance between patients with nonulcer IC and women without bladder symptoms about to undergo tubal ligation [12].

8.2 Histopathology in Bladder Pain Syndrome/Interstitial Cystitis—General

The role of histopathology in the diagnosis of Bladder Pain Syndrome/Interstitial Cystitis (BPS/IC) is primarily one of excluding other possible diagnoses. Possible confusing and potentially harmful conditions must be ruled out; carcinoma and carcinoma in situ, eosinophilic cystitis, tuberculous cystitis, as well as any other entities with a specific tissue diagnosis, such as enteric metaplasia, cystitis glandularis, squamous cell metaplasia and nephrogenic metaplasia. Some of these metaplastic conditions have malignant counterparts and in order to rule out such possible malignancies, deep bladder biopsies and sometimes directed immunohistochemical staining may be necessary.

However, biopsy retrieval and histopathological examination may also be of value when it comes to diagnosing BPS/IC. Even though most histopathologic features are not distinctive of BPS/IC in nonulcer disease, certain signs are, for practical clinical purposes, patognomonic for classic IC. In recent decades, understanding of the properties of various cell system has developed dramatically and, moreover, the diagnosis with standard staining procedures and light microscopy can now be further refined with immunohistochemistry and even more sophisticated and sensitive amplification techniques such as in situ hybridization, polymerase chain reaction and various blot and array techniques.

8.3 Biopsy Retrieval, Fixation, and Staining Procedures

To facilitate the possibility for a correct histopathological diagnosis of BPS/IC, biopsies should be obtained by transurethral resection of large strips of the bladder wall, including the detrusor muscle; however cold cup biopsies can also be a feasible option. This is somewhat depending on local tradition but the choice of biopsy retrieval technique can also be governed by which kind of pathology is suspected and what pathology the clinician finds important to rule out.

Formaldehyde fixation (4%, 10%) is mandatory and fixation rate is approximately 1 mm per hour; hence small biopsies are fixated by the time they reach the pathology department. In the laboratory the specimen is dehydrated, paraffin or wax embedded, and cut into series of 4 μm sections. The specimen is thereafter deparaffinized and stained with hematoxylin/eosin (Htx-Eo) prior to dehydration and mounting with coverslips. Additional stainings are often performed in order to guide the pathologist into a more correct diagnosis. For instance Van Gieson or Sitius may be helpful to demonstrate fibrosis. Most antibodies are tested on formaldehyde-fixated tissue and mast cell tryptase may nowadays be visualised using a specific antibody. Toluidin Blue, a metachromatic dye, may be used to stain mast cells but the staining procedure with Toluidin blue is problematic. The method is very dependent on low pH during which circumstances mast cells containing heparin and chondroitin-sulfate are visualized. Chemicals like HCl, citronic acid, and the dye Toludin blue is unhealthy for the personnel handling the dying process. This method has now been replaced with a mast cell tryptase antibody (Fig. 8.1).

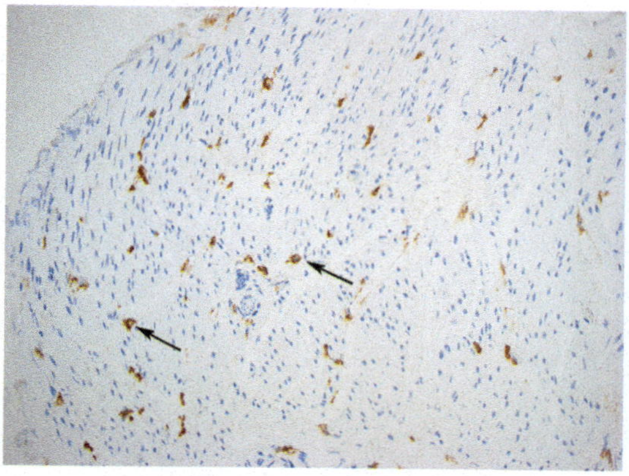

Fig. 8.1 The detrusor muscle. Tryptase in mast cells visualized by immunohistochemistry. Mastocytosis with a relatively high number of mast cells within the muscle bundle (*arrows*), in this case >50 per mm^2, Htx/eo

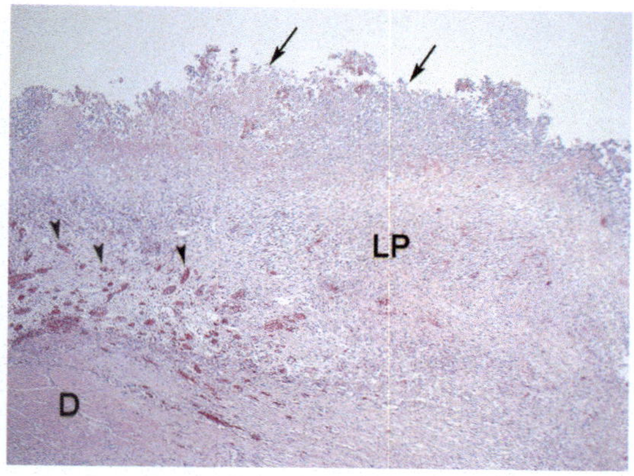

Fig. 8.3 Abnormal bladder. Severe case of bladder pain syndrome. Epithelial denudation, ulceration with fibrin and inflammatory cells (*arrows*). Granulation formation (*arrowheads*) in lamina propria (LP) reaching deeper portions and the detrusor muscle compartments (D), Htx/eo

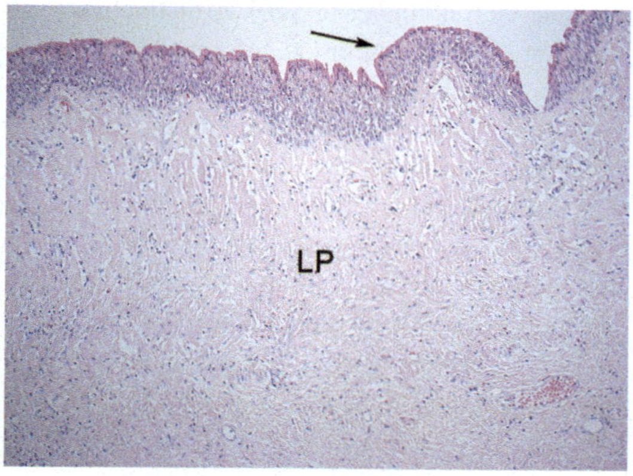

Fig. 8.2 Normal bladder. Intact urothelium with umbella cells (*arrow*). Beneath the urothelium resides the lamina propria (LP), Htx/eo

8.4 Light Microscopic Features

Specimens from patients with BPS/IC type 3C (classic IC) as a rule display striking histologic alterations from normal mucosa (Fig. 8.2), with prominent ulcerations that may be covered by fibrin mixed with inflammatory cells, in particular neutrophils (Fig. 8.3). The ulcerations are often wedge shaped and involve the superficial part of the lamina propria, not seldom extending all the way into the lamina muscularis mucosae. Underlying granulation tissue is present in the vast majority of the subjects [13]. These findings tally with those reported already 100 years ago by Hunner, who reported the abundance of granulation tissue formation as well as chronic inflammation involving all coats of the bladder [14]. There is an abnormal microvascularity in the lamina propria which may result in petechial bleeding or glomerulations, and possibly also ulceration as a consequence of ischemia, this in turn may bring about hemorrhage in the entire lamina propria. BPS/IC type 3C (classic IC) hence displays marked inflammatory changes in the lamina propria, including the presence of lymphocytes, plasma cells, mast cells and neutrophils. Eosinophils are generally few. Germinal centre formation may be seen. Fibrosis is commonly displayed in BPS/IC and especially inter and intra lamellar fibrosis in the detrusor muscle should be evaluated and reported (Fig. 8.4a, b).

The counting of mast cells in the detrusor muscle, using a grid, is mandatory in diagnosing BPS/IC. The mast cell count is usually high above 25 per mm^2 (Fig. 8.1).

The aforementioned light microscopic features differ markedly from what can be seen in nonulcer IC. Lepinard reported that whereas pancystitis affected the three layers of bladder wall, this was not the case in nonulcerative disease [15]. In another report, comprising 64 patients with ulcerative disease and 44 with nonulcerative IC, ulcerative disease had mucosal ulceration and

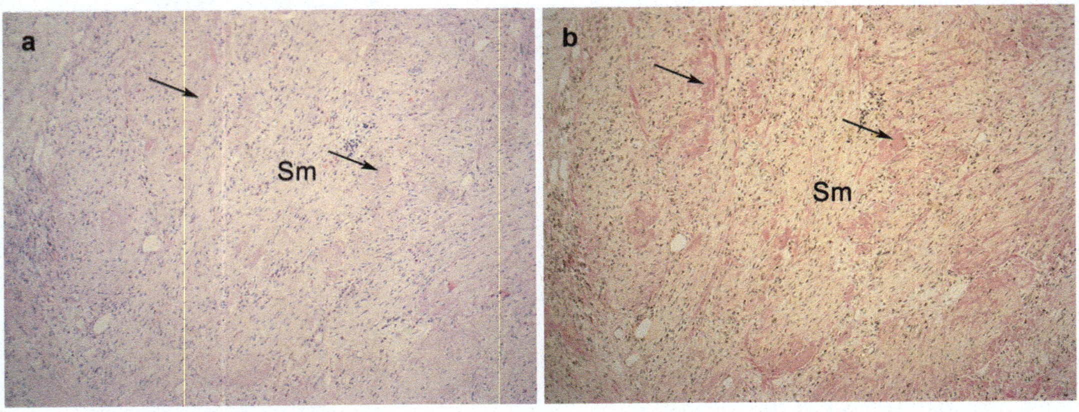

Fig. 8.4 The detrusor muscle with smooth muscle (Sm) and intralamellar fibroses (*arrows*). (**a**) Htx/eosin. (**b**) Van Gieson staining, high lightening the fibroses in between the smooth muscle bundles as pink aggregates

hemorrhage, granulation tissue, severe inflammatory infiltrates, high mast cell counts, and perineural infiltrates. The nonulcer group, despite sharing a similar sympomatology and the same chronic course, had an impervious mucosa with a meagre inflammatory response, the main feature being numerous, mucosal ruptures and suburothelial hemorrhages [16]. Not seldom, biopsies can be perfectly normal in nonulcer IC.

8.5 Ultrastructural Studies

Electron microscopy has not been very successful in diagnosing BPS/IC. In an early paper on this topic, Collan et al. stated that there was a considerable similarity of the ultrastructure of epithelial cells between controls and IC patients [17], and some 10 years later Dixon et al. also failed to discover any differences in the morphologic appearances of urothelial cells in patients with IC as compared to controls [18]. Neither could Anderström et al. see any unambiguous ultrastructural surface characteristics for IC, however, the proportion of cells covered by round, uniform and pleomorphic microvilli was higher in the IC patients than in controls [19].

At variance with these reports on lack of diagnostic positive histopathologic signs in nonulcer IC, Elbadawi and Light concluded that ultrastructural changes appear to be sufficiently distinctive to be diagnostic in specimens submitted for pathologic confirmation of nonulcer interstitial cystitis. They performed a detailed ultrastructural study on patients with nonulcer IC [20]. A distinctive combination of peculiar muscle cell profiles, injury of intrinsic vessels and nerves in muscularis and suburothelium, and discohesive urothelium was observed in lesional and less markedly in nonlesional samples of all specimens. Marked edema of various tissue elements and cells appeared to be a common denominator of many observed changes. Urothelial changes disrupted the true permeability barrier. Neural changes included a combination of degenerative and regenerative features.

8.6 Histopathological Detection of Mast Cells in BPS/IC

Mast cells are regarded not only as cells involved in allergic tissue reactions but as multifunctional immunocompetent cells involved in a variety of tissue reactions such as chronic inflammation, examples of which are classic IC and rheumatoid arthritis as well as fibrosis [21]. It has thus been shown that the mast cell, in addition to histamine and heparin, also contains other highly potent inflammatory mediators such as leucotrienes, cytokines and the angiogenic and fibroblast stimulatory factor bFGF (basic fibroblast growth factor) [22, 23]. In addition to allergen binding, nerve-derived mediators may also stimulate mast cell secretion. Several lines of evidence support the concept of a neuroimmune connection [24] and morphological association between mast cells and neuropeptide-containing nerves has been demonstrated [25–27].

It was demonstrated, in bladder specimens from patients with classic IC, non-ulcer IC and controls, that mast cells were visualised in terms of metachromasia, reflecting glycosaminoglycan content, and immunohistochemically, visualising tryptase, chymase and IL-6 as well as the surface markers CD 117 and stem cell factor (SCF) [28]. In this report, classic IC displayed a 6–10-fold increase of mast cells in terms of proteinase positivity while nonulcer IC revealed twice as many mast cells as controls. In contrast to non-ulcer IC and controls, classic IC displayed an abundance of epithelial mast cells.

8.7 Histopathological Detection of Immunocompetent Cells in BPS/IC

There are numerous reports on autoantibodies in patients with IC [29–31] and, moreover, some of the common clinical and histopathological characteristics present in IC patients show certain similarities with other known autoimmune phenomena. This is the background to the theory that IC may arise from autoimmune disturbances. The role of autoimmunity in IC is controversial and the disease is not thought to originate from a direct autoimmune attack on the bladder. Rather, some of the autoimmune symptoms and pathologic findings in IC arise indirectly as a result of tissue destruction and inflammation from other, as yet unknown, causes.

In a study of 47 IC patients, Mattila et al. found immune deposits in the vessel walls of 33 patients [32] and in a subsequent study, electron microscopy evidence of endothelial injury was found in 14 out of 20 IC patients [33]. There is, no doubt, an inflammatory response in classic IC, of a chronic nature, and this makes it possible that there is a cell-mediated autoimmune response at hand. In a report encompassing 24 classic IC patients, nine nonulcer patients and ten controls [34] it was found that the classic IC patients displayed aggregates of T-cells as well as B-nodules with focal germinal centres. There was a decreased or normal helper/suppressor ratio and suppressor cytotoxic cells were present in the germinal centres. The nonulcer patients, conversely, had only slightly increased numbers of lymphoid cells, dominated by T-helper cells, the nonulcer group not differing significantly from the controls.

In the very recent publication by Maeda et al. patients with Hunner type interstitial cystitis (HIC) and non-Hunner type interstitial cystitis (NHIC) were compared [35]. Using immunohistochemical quantification of infiltrating T-lymphocytes, B-lymphocytes and plasma cells, the authors were able to demonstrate that lymphoplasmacytic infiltration was significantly more severe in HIC specimens than in NHIC specimens. They moreover disclosed that the loss of residual epithelium was considerably decreased in HIC specimens but not in NHIC specimens. Finally, in situ hybridization of the light chains was performed to examine clonal B-cell expansion and the authors demonstrated that such expansion of light-chain-restricted B-cells was observed in 31% of cases of HIC. The authors concluded that NHIC and HIC appear to be divergent pathological entities, the latter being characterized by pancystitis, frequent clonal B-cell expansion and epithelial denudation. The very same research group also used double-immunofluorescence for CXCR3 and CD138 to detect CXCR3 expression in plasma cells from subjects with HIC and NHIC, respectively. Correlations between CXCR3 positivity and lymphocytic and plasma cell numbers and clinical parameters were explored. The density of CXCR3-positive cells showed no significant differences between HIC and non-IC cystitis specimens. However, distribution of CXCR3-positivity in plasma cells indicated co-localization of CXCR3 with CD138 in HIC specimens, but not in non-IC cystitis specimens [36].

8.8 Nitric Oxide Evaporation and iNOS Expression in BPS/IC

Recent research by us and by others has suggested that nitric oxide (NO) metabolism might play an important role in this context, the luminal production of NO being high in HIC but not in NHIC [37, 38]. Moreover, inducible nitric oxide synthase (iNOS) has been demonstrated to be abundant, in the urothelium and in inflammatory cells in patients with HIC, not only by immunohistochemistry but also on the transcriptional level [39, 40].

Acknowledgments We would like to thank Ulric Pedersen for his contribution to the preparation of included figures.

References

1. Skene AJC. Diseases of bladder and urethra in women. New York: Wm Wood; 1887. p. 167.
2. Hunner GL. A rare type of bladder ulcer in women; report of cases. Boston Med Surg J. 1915;172:660–4.
3. Hand JR. Interstitial cystitis: report of 223 cases (204 women and 19 men). J Urol. 1949;61:291–310.
4. Messing EM, Stamey TA. Interstitial cystitis: early diagnosis, pathology and treatment. Urology. 1978;12:381–92.
5. Fall M, Johansson SL, Aldenborg F. Chronic interstitial cystitis: a heterogeneous syndrome. J Urol. 1987;137(1):35–8.
6. Koziol JA, Adams HP, Frutos A. Discrimination between the ulcerous and the nonulcerous forms of interstitial cystitis by noninvasive findings. J Urol. 1996;155(1):87–90.
7. Logadottir Y, Fall M, Kabjorn-Gustafsson C, Peeker R. Clinical characteristics differ considerably between phenotypes of bladder pain syndrome/interstitial cystitis. Scand J Urol Nephrol. 2012;46(5):365–70.
8. Peeker R, Fall M. Toward a precise definition of interstitial cystitis: further evidence of differences in classic and nonulcer disease. J Urol. 2002;167(6):2470–2.
9. Killinger KA, Boura JA, Peters KM. Pain in interstitial cystitis/bladder pain syndrome: do characteristics differ in ulcerative and non-ulcerative subtypes? Int Urogynecol J. 2013;24(8):1295–301.
10. Peters KM, Killinger KA, Mounayer MH, Boura JA. Are ulcerative and nonulcerative interstitial cystitis/painful bladder syndrome 2 distinct diseases? A study of coexisting conditions. Urology. 2011;78(2):301–8.
11. Parsons CL. Interstitial cystitis: clinical manifestations and diagnostic criteria in over 200 cases. Neurourol Urodyn. 1990;9:241–50.
12. Waxman JA, Sulak PJ, Kuehl TJ. Cystoscopic findings consistent with interstitial cystitis in normal women undergoing tubal ligation. J Urol. 1998;160(5):1663–7.
13. Johansson SL, Ogawa K, Fall M. The pathology of interstitial cystitis. In: Sant GR, editor. Interstitial cystitis. Philadelphia: Lippincott-Raven; 1997. p. 143–52.
14. Hunner GL. A rare type of bladder ulcer: further notes, with a report of eighteen cases. JAMA. 1918;70:203–12.
15. Lepinard V. Interstitial cystitis. Ann Urol (Paris). 1998;32(6–7):349–51.
16. Johansson SL, Fall M. Clinical features and spectrum of light microscopic changes in interstitial cystitis. J Urol. 1990;143(6):1118–24.
17. Collan Y, Alfthan O, Kivilaakso E, Oravisto KJ. Electron microscopic and histological findings on urinary bladder epithelium in interstitial cystitis. Eur Urol. 1976;2(5):242–7.
18. Dixon J, Holm-Bentzen M, Gilpin C. Electron microscopic investigation of the bladder urothelium and glycocalyx in patients with interstitial cystitis. J Urol. 1986;135:621–5.
19. Anderstrom CR, Fall M, Johansson SL. Scanning electron microscopic findings in interstitial cystitis. Br J Urol. 1989;63(3):270–5.
20. Elbadawi A, Light JK. Distinctive ultrastructural pathology of nonulcerative interstitial cystitis. Urol Int. 1996;56:137–62.
21. Hunt LW, Colby TV, Weiler DA, Sur S, Butterfield JH. Immunofluorescent staining for mast cells in idiopathic pulmonary fibrosis: quantification and evidence for extracellular release of mast cell tryptase. Mayo Clin Proc. 1992;67(10):941–8.
22. Qu Z, Liebler JM, Powers MR, Galey T, Ahmadi P, Huang XN, et al. Mast cells are a major source of basic fibroblast growth factor in chronic inflammation and cutaneous hemangioma. Am J Pathol. 1995;147:564–73.
23. Stevens LR, Austen KF. Recent advances in the cellular and molecular biology of mast cells. Immunol Today. 1989;10:381–6.
24. Williams RM, Bienenstock J, Stead RH. Mast cells: the neuroimmune connection. Chem Immunol. 1995;61:208–35.
25. Keith IM, Jin J, Saban R. Nerve-mast cell interaction in normal guinea pig urinary bladder. J Comp Neurol. 1995;363(1):28–36.
26. Naukkarinen A, Harvima IT, Aalto ML, Harvima RJ, Horsmanheimo M. Quantitative analysis of contact sites between mast cells and sensory nerves in cutaneous psoriasis and lichen planus based on a histochemical double staining technique. Arch Dermatol Res. 1991;283(7):433–7.
27. Newson B, Dahlstrom A, Enerback L, Ahlman H. Suggestive evidence for a direct innervation of mucosal mast cells. Neuroscience. 1983;10(2):565–70.
28. Peeker R, Enerbäck L, Fall M, Aldenborg F. Recruitment, distribution and phenotypes of mast cells in interstitial cystitis. J Urol. 2000; 163:1009–15.
29. Ochs RL, Stein T Jr, Peebles CL, Gittes RF, Tan EM. Autoantibodies in interstitial cystitis. J Urol. 1994;151(3):587–92.
30. Oravisto KJ. Interstitial cystitis as an autoimmune disease. A review. Eur Urol. 1980;6:10–3.
31. Silk MR. Bladder antibodies in interstitial cystitis. J Urol. 1970;103:307–9.
32. Mattila J, Pitkanen R, Vaalasti T, Seppanen J. Fine-structural evidence for vascular injury in patients

with interstitial cystitis. Virchows Arch A Pathol Anat Histopathol. 1983;398(3):347–55.

33. Tan EM. Antinuclear antibodies: diagnostic markers for autoimmune diseases and probes for cell biology. Adv Immunol. 1989;44:93–151.
34. Harrington DS, Fall M, Johansson SL. Interstitial cystitis: bladder mucosa lymphocyte immunophenotyping and peripheral blood flow cytometry analysis. J Urol. 1990;144(4):868–71.
35. Maeda D, Akiyama Y, Morikawa T, Kunita A, Ota Y, Katoh H, et al. Hunner-type (classic) interstitial cystitis: a distinct inflammatory disorder characterized by pancystitis, with frequent expansion of clonal B-cells and epithelial denudation. PLoS One. 2015;10(11):e0143316.
36. Akiyama Y, Morikawa T, Maeda D, Shintani Y, Niimi A, Nomiya A, et al. Increased CXCR3 expression of infiltrating plasma cells in hunner type interstitial cystitis. Sci Rep. 2016;6:28652.
37. Ehren I, Hosseini A, Herulf M, Lundberg JO, Wiklund NP. Measurement of luminal nitric oxide in bladder inflammation using a silicon balloon catheter: a novel minimally invasive method. Urology. 1999; 54:264–7.
38. Logadottir Y, Ehren I, Fall M, Wiklund NP, Peeker R. Intravesical nitric oxide production discriminates between classic and nonulcer interstitial cystitis. J Urol. 2004;171:1148–50.
39. Koskela LR, Thiel T, Ehren I, De Verdier PJ, Wiklund NP. Localization and expression of inducible nitric oxide synthase in biopsies from patients with interstitial cystitis. J Urol. 2008;180:737–41.
40. Logadottir Y, Hallsberg L, Fall M, Peeker R, Delbro D. Bladder pain syndrome/interstitial cystitis ESSIC type 3C: high expression of inducible nitric oxide synthase in inflammatory cells. Scand J Urol. 2013;47:52–6.

Mast Cells and Interstitial Cystitis

9

Frank Aldenborg, Magnus Fall, and Lennart Enerbäck

Mast cells (MC) are tissue-resident immune cells that participate in first line host defense, responding to allergic challenge and pathogen attacks. Following appropriate stimulation they release immuno-modulators, and vaso- and neuroactive compounds. Early reports suggest that MCs are innervated [1] and their anatomical proximity to vasculature and nerve fibers underpin the likelihood of functioning neuro-immune interfaces. The biological role of MCs is diversified.

MCs have been in the focus of interstitial cystitis research for a long time and it has been repeatedly suggested that histo-pathologic demonstration of MC hyperplasia represents a momentous diagnostic tool. In the 80-ties the critical number of 28 MCs/mm^2 was by many suggested as *the* proof of the diagnosis [2, 3]. It has to be remembered, though, that MC counts in the specimen of bladder mucosa and detrusor muscle does not disclose the absolute number of cells residing in the biopsy. Certainly, the degree of MC expansion is determinative but laboratory techniques have a considerable impact as to numbers, too. During the last decades, there has been a significant development of technologies resulting in increasing accuracy of MC demonstration. Naphtolesterase staining [2] was replaced by the more sensitive toluidine blue staining, reinforced by more appropriate fixation techniques to overcome blocking of dye-binding [4, 5]. Currently, immunohistochemical tryptase labeling has been found superior and more robust comparing to earlier methods [6, 7] and is the method recommended today [8].

9.1 What Did We Get Right?

The dramatic increase of MC counts in classic IC [5, 7], (ESSIC type 3) [9] compared to non-Hunner subjects and controls emphasize the fundamental difference between phenotypes with and without Hunner lesions.

9.2 What Seminal Publications Changed Our Thinking?

Certainly, MCs is one of the key players in classic IC/BPS (ESSIC 3C) and the reports from the 80-ties directed an attention to these cells [2, 3], an important attention. The rare finding in human biology of transepithelial MC migration demonstrated in classic IC [5, 7], with connection to the IgE system, among other things indicated that an

F. Aldenborg • L. Enerbäck
Department of Pathology, Sahlgrenska Academy at the University of Gothenburg, SE-41345 Göteborg, Sweden

M. Fall, M.D., Ph.D. (✉)
Department of Urology, Institute of Clinical Sciences, Sahlgrenska Academy at the University of Gothenburg, SE-41345 Göteborg, Sweden
e-mail: magnus.fall@urology.gu.se

P.M. Hanno et al. (eds.), *Bladder Pain Syndrome – An Evolution*,
https://doi.org/10.1007/978-3-319-61449-6_9

allergic response could come into question but if so, what is the agent? The etiology and pathogenesis of BPS/IC is still not resolved and MCs may hold one of the keys.

9.3 Where Were We Off Base?

MC counts in a specimen of bladder mucosa and detrusor muscle do not disclose the absolute number of cells residing in the tissue. A number of factors govern the counts found in a biopsy and it is not possible to establish a fixed critical number. Fortunately, tryptase techniques have made comparison between different laboratories more reliable, though.

9.4 Where Do We Go from Here?

Although the disease mechanisms in BPS/IC and the role of MCs certainly are complex [10] and partly difficult to grasp, one capacity of particular interest is that MC can modulate synaptic responses. Further, MC-mediated pain can be disease-specific [11], features clearly motivating a continued interest of MCs in BPS/IC.

The cell components in classic IC (ESSIC type 3C) include lymphocytes, plasma cells, granulocytes, macrophages and mast cells [12, 13], and this characteristic combination of cell elements has something to tell. There is a documented interplay between MCs and T-lymphocytes; interactions between the various cell components present in the infiltrate has to be expected. Thorough analysis of biological possibilities related to the features of the inflammatory infiltrate might give clues to development of rational pharmacologic treatment.

References

1. Newson B, Dahlstrom A, Enerback L, Ahlman H. Suggestive evidence for a direct innervation of mucosal mast cells. Neuroscience. 1983;10(2):565–70.
2. Larsen S, Thompson SA, Hald T, Barnard RJ, Gilpin CJ, Dixon JS, et al. Mast cells in interstitial cystitis. Br J Urol. 1982;54(3):283–6.
3. Kastrup J, Hald T, Larsen S, Nielsen VG. Histamine content and mast cell count of detrusor muscle in patients with interstitial cystitis and other types of chronic cystitis. Br J Urol. 1983;55(5):495–500.
4. Enerbäck L. Mast cells in rat gastrointestinal mucosa. I. Effect of fixation. Acta Pathol Microbiol Scand. 1966;66:289–302.
5. Aldenborg F, Fall M, Enerbäck L. Proliferation and transepithelial migration of mucosal mast cells in interstitial cystitis. Immunology. 1986;58:411–6.
6. Irani A-MA, Bradford TR, Kepley CL, Schechter NM, Schwartz LB. Detection of MCT and MCTC types of human mast cells by immunohistochemistry using new monoclonal anti-tryptase and anti-chymase antibodies. J Histochem Cytochem. 1989;37:1509–15.
7. Peeker R, Fall M, Enerbäck L, Aldenborg F. Recruitment, distribution and phenotypes of mast cells in interstitial cystitis. J Urol. 2000;163:1009–15.
8. Larsen M, Mortensen S, Nordling J, Horn T. Quantifying mast cells in bladder pain syndrome by immunohistochemical analysis. BJU Int. 2008;102:204–7.
9. van de Merwe JP, Nordling J, Bouchelouche P, Bouchelouche K, Cervigni M, Daha LK, et al. Diagnostic criteria, classification, and nomenclature for painful bladder syndrome/interstitial cystitis: an ESSIC proposal. Eur Urol. 2008;53(1):60–7.
10. Theoarides TC, Pang X, Letourneau R, Sant GR. Interstitial cystitis: a neuroimmunoendocrine disorder. Ann N Y Acad Sci. 1998;840:619–34.
11. Aich A, Afrin L, Gupta K. Mast cell-mediated mechanisms of nociception. Int J Mol Sci. 2015;4(16):29069–92.
12. Fall M, Johansson SL, Vahlne A. A clinicopathological and virological study of interstitial cystitis. J Urol. 1985;133(5):771–3.
13. Johansson SL, Fall M. Clinical features and spectrum of light microscopic changes in interstitial cystitis. J Urol. 1990;143(6):1118–24.

10 Mast Cells as Biomarkers for Bladder Pain Syndrome/Interstitial Cystitis?

Marianne Gamper, Sigrid Regauer, and Volker Viereck

Abstract

Results of mast cell staining in early and recent studies agree surprisingly well, even though different staining methods have been applied. Increased mast cell counts in subepithelial tissue and in the detrusor muscle are characteristic for bladder pain syndrome/interstitial cystitis (BPS/IC) with Hunner's lesion, or "classic interstitial cystitis", but not for BPS/IC without Hunner's lesion or overactive bladder syndrome (OAB). BPS/IC without Hunner's lesion and OAB cannot be differentiated by mast cell counts, activation or localization. Recent studies found that mast cell evaluation is not necessary for the diagnosis of BPS/IC, especially because cystoscopy is sufficient to identify BPS/IC with Hunner's lesion. Other histological markers, such as a defective urothelium, the presence of lymphocytic infiltration/lymphocyte aggregates and submucosal sensory hyperinnervation are better criteria to distinguish BPS/IC without Hunner's lesion from OAB. The origin of BPS/IC still remains unknown. Future goals should include the identification of early disease forms and adequate therapies to prevent disease progression. Objective, reliable and preferentially non-invasive markers for diagnosis and treatment monitoring have to be determined.

Keywords

Mast cells • Diagnosis • Histopathology • Immunohistochemistry • Toluidine blue staining

M. Gamper (✉) • V. Viereck
Department of Gynecology and Obstetrics, Cantonal Hospital Frauenfeld,
CH-8501 Frauenfeld, Switzerland
e-mail: marianne.gamper@stgag.ch; volker.viereck@stgag.ch

S. Regauer
Institute of Pathology, Medical University Graz,
A-8036 Graz, Austria
e-mail: sigrid.regauer@medunigraz.at

10.1 Introduction

Thirty years ago, diagnosis of the then called "classic interstitial cystitis" was based on the symptoms chronic pain and urinary frequency, the presence of Hunner's lesion in cystoscopy and inflammation in biopsy. Later, some guidelines recommended diagnosis solely based on symptoms while cystoscopy and bladder biopsy

P.M. Hanno et al. (eds.), *Bladder Pain Syndrome – An Evolution*,
https://doi.org/10.1007/978-3-319-61449-6_10

were facultative [1]. But different classification systems and nomenclature made comparison between studies especially difficult. Today, the circle is closing and cystoscopy and bladder biopsy regain significance for the diagnosis [2].

10.2 The Technique of Tissue Fixation and Mast Cell Staining in the Late 1980s

In the late 1980s, chemical staining with toluidine blue, but not immunohistochemistry with anti-mast cell tryptase antibodies, was the standard histopathological technique to detect mast cells. Hence, the optimization of staining and fixation methods was prominently discussed in the book chapter by Aldenborg et al. The authors found two types of mast cells in the bladder wall of "classic interstitial cystitis". One type was predominant in the submucosa and could not be visualized after routine 4% formaldehyde fixation, but needed a special fixation technique, e.g. with 0.6% formaldehyde/ 0.5% acetic acid. The other type was predominant in the detrusor muscle and needed no special fixation for detection [3]. Submucosal and epithelial mast cell numbers were twofold higher for patients with "classic interstitial cystitis" than for healthy controls, but detection was only possible after the special fixation with formaldehyde/acetic acid. With routine formaldehyde fixation, only a twofold increase in detrusor mast cell counts could be seen. The authors conclude that mast cell proliferation and migration towards the periphery and the epithelium of the bladder wall is characteristic for "classic interstitial cystitis".

The ESSIC classified types of bladder pain syndrome/interstitial cystitis (BPS/IC) based on cystoscopy and biopsy findings [4]. Interestingly, "detrusor mastocytosis" per se, defined as >28 mast cells/mm^2, can assign a biopsy to the most severe category C [5]. This number was not referenced in this meeting's proceedings and most likely originated from an early study by Larsen et al. [6], before Aldenborg et al. described the above mentioned special fixation method to additionally stain submucosal mast cells [3]. Thus, current guidelines concentrate on detrusor mast cell counts presumably because a publication with outdated fixation and staining techniques was considered.

10.3 Mast Cell Staining 30 Years Later

Today, immunohistochemistry with antibodies against mast cell tryptase is the gold standard for mast cell staining. This technique was shown to be equivalent or superior to toluidine staining [7]. In a recent study with 56 patients [8], subepithelial mast cell localization was predominantly found for BPS/IC with Hunner's lesion (Fig. 10.1b), but not for BPS/IC without Hunner's lesion, overactive bladder (OAB) and healthy controls. This result thus agrees with the above described findings by Aldenborg et al. Detrusor mast cell counts were slightly elevated in BPS/IC with Hunner's lesion. The calculated optimal cut-off value to predict BPS/IC with Hunner's lesion was 32 mast cells/mm^2, and thus, close to the threshold number of 28 mast cells/mm^2 [4]. But this number only achieved 68% accuracy and a 38% positive prediction value, and therefore detrusor mast cell counts cannot be considered a reliable diagnostic criterion. Furthermore, BPS/IC without Hunner's lesion and OAB cannot be distinguished by detrusor mast cell numbers, and biopsies often did not include sufficient amounts of detrusor muscle for a thorough evaluation [5]. In addition, submucosal mast cell counts and the presence of mast cell activation, defined by degranulation (= location of granules outside the cytoplasm, Fig. 10.1c), were poor diagnostic criteria; no significant differences were found between patient subgroups. Intraepithelial mast cells were present in only two cases of BPS/IC with Hunner's lesion (12.5%), while often, the urothelium was absent or defective. This is in contrast to Aldenborg et al. that frequently detected intraepithelial mast cells (94%) [3].

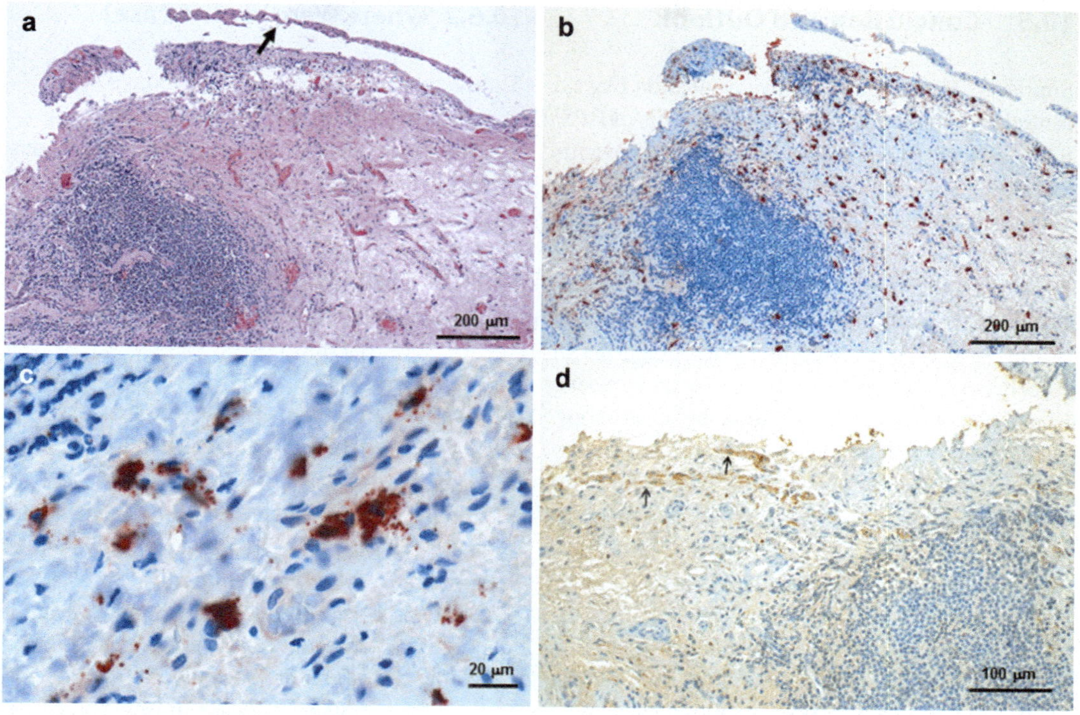

Fig. 10.1 Bladder biopsy of a patient with BPS/IC with Hunner's lesion, lesional area. (**a**) Hematoxylin and eosin staining shows an area of erosion with detachment of the urothelium (*arrow*) from the submucosa. Underneath the ulcer bed, the blood vessels in the submucosa are distended and filled with erythrocytes. A large nodular lymphocytic aggregate can be seen on the left. (**b**) Immunohistochemistry with an antibody against mast cell tryptase shows numerous mast cells (in *red*) in subepithelial localization and throughout the submucosa. Note the sparing of the lymphocytic infiltrate. (**c**) Mast cells show some degree of degranulation, with the majority of granules localized inside the cytoplasm surrounding the nucleus and with a few granules outside the cell (= sign of activation, *red small dots*). (**d**) Immunohistochemistry with an antibody against PGP9.5 stains sensory nerve fibers (in *brown*, *arrows*) in the ulcer bed

10.4 Biopsy Evaluation for the Diagnosis of BPS/IC

Other histopathological criteria turned out to be better markers for the diagnosis of BPS/IC [9]. Dense to medium lymphocytic infiltrates, frequently combined with the presence of nodular lymphocyte aggregates (Fig. 10.1a) or lymph follicles were characteristic for BPS/IC with and without Hunner's lesion, with 86% accuracy and an 85% positive prediction value. Also an absent or defective urothelium (Fig. 10.1a) was a strong criterion for separating BPS/IC from OAB, with 88% accuracy and an 83% positive prediction value. Moreover, immunohistochemical staining with antibodies to PGP9.5, a marker for unmyelinated nociceptive sensory nerve fibers, showed submucosal sensory hyperinnervation (Fig. 10.1d) in cases of BPS/IC, but not in OAB, with 88% accuracy and an 83% positive prediction value. Typically, these nerve fibers are not present in the submucosa of healthy patients, but under pathological conditions they proliferate, partly under the influence of neurotrophins, such as nerve growth factor (NGF). Immunohistochemical staining of the NGF-receptor $p75^{NTR}$ in basal urothelial cells was a sign for urothelial regeneration and thus a further evidence for BPS/IC.

10.5 Conclusion and Outlook

Similar to 30 years ago, biopsy evaluation plays a central and important role for the diagnosis of BPS/IC. Mast cell hyperplasia and migration towards the ulcer bed or beneath the epithelium were evidently characteristic for BPS/IC with Hunner's lesion. BPS/IC without Hunner's lesion and OAB, however, could not be distinguished by mast cell counts, activation or localization. Therefore, mast cell evaluation is not helpful for the diagnosis of BPS/IC, especially because BPS/IC with Hunner's lesion can already be identified by cystoscopy. Other histological features, such as the sensory hyperinnervation, urothelial defects and lymphocytic infiltration are better histopathological criteria to differentiate between BPS/IC and OAB.

The origin of BPS/IC still remains unknown. Thirty years ago, Aldenborg et al. ended their article by suggesting an infection or an allergic reaction as possible causes. These assumptions still remain valid, and very likely, causes are multifactorial. To find out, further studies are required. Research will also focus on the identification and adequate therapy of early forms to prevent disease progression. A good diagnosis and treatment monitoring, e.g. based on robust objective histopathological markers, is mandatory to achieve these goals.

10.6 Questions

10.6.1 What Did We Get Right?

Thirty years ago:

- Assessment of bladder biopsies for diagnosis of BPS/IC.
- The finding that mast cell proliferation and migration towards the periphery and the epithelium of the bladder wall is characteristic for "classic interstitial cystitis".

10.6.2 Where Were We Off Base?

Time between 30 years ago and today:

- To define detrusor mastocytosis (>28 mast cells/mm^2) per se as a criterion to assign a biopsy to the most severe category C (ESSIC).
- To base this criterion on a publication with outdated fixation and staining techniques.

10.6.3 What Seminal Publications Changed Our Thinking?

- Immunohistochemistry with antibodies against mast cell tryptase was equivalent or superior to toluidine staining [7].
- Detrusor mast cell counts were not a reliable diagnostic criterion for BPS/IC with Hunner's lesion, and often, biopsies did not include sufficient amounts of detrusor muscle for a thorough evaluation [8].
- BPS/IC without Hunner's lesion and OAB could not be distinguished by mast cell counts, activation or localization [8].
- BPS/IC and OAB can be distinguished by sensory hyperinnervation, urothelial defects and lymphocytic infiltration [9].

10.6.4 Where Do We Go from Here?

- Use new molecular markers for the diagnosis of BPS/IC (biopsies, urine).
- To find out if non-lesional forms of BPS/IC are early forms or pre-stages of BPS/IC with Hunner's lesion and to define targeted therapies to prevent disease progression.
- To identify the origin of BPS/IC and to apply causal therapies.

References

1. Hanno PM, Burks DA, Clemens JQ, Dmochowski RR, Erickson D, FitzGerald MP, et al. Diagnosis and treatment of interstitial cystitis/bladder pain syndrome. American Urological Association (AUA) guideline. 2014:1–45.
2. Belknap S, Blalock, E, Erickson D. The challenges of interstitial cystitis: current status and future prospects. Drugs 2015;75:2057–63.
3. Aldenborg F, Fall M, Enerback L. Proliferation and transepithelial migration of mucosal mast cells in interstitial cystitis. Immunology. 1986;58:411–6.
4. van de Merwe JP, Nordling J, Bouchelouche P, Bouchelouche K, Cervigni M, Daha LK, et al. Diagnostic criteria, classification, and nomenclature for painful bladder syndrome/interstitial cystitis: an ESSIC proposal. Eur Urol. 2008;53:60–7.
5. Nordling J, Anjum FH, Bade JJ, Bouchelouche K, Bouchelouche P, Cervigni M, et al. Primary evaluation of patients suspected of having interstitial cystitis (IC). Eur Urol. 2004;45:662–9.
6. Larsen S, Thompson SA, Hald T, Barnard RJ, Gilpin CJ, Dixon JS, et al. Mast cells in interstitial cystitis. Br J Urol. 1982;54:283–6.
7. Yamada T, Murayama T, Mita H, Akiyama K. Subtypes of bladder mast cells in interstitial cystitis. Int J Urol. 2000;7:292–7.
8. Gamper M, Regauer S, Welter J, Eberhard J, Viereck V. Are mast cells still good biomarkers for bladder pain syndrome/interstitial cystitis? J Urol. 2015;193:1994–2000.
9. Regauer S, Gamper M, Fehr MK, Viereck V. Sensory hyperinnervation distinguishes bladder pain syndrome/interstitial cystitis from overactive bladder syndrome. J Urol. 2017;197:159–66.

11 Diagnosis of Interstitial Cystitis: A Clinical, Endoscopic and Pathologic Approach

Joop P. van de Merwe

11.1 What Did We Get Right?

Criteria for the diagnosis of a disease are needed if the disease may be confused with other diseases due to overlapping features. This was clearly the case for interstitial cystitis (IC) 30 years ago. Therefore, the National Institute of Diabetes and Digestive and Kidney Disease (NIDDK) formulated criteria for diagnosis in 1987 [1]. The NIDDK criteria were specifically designed for research. For research purposes, most scientists will only accept "certain" diagnoses. Consequently, patients had to fulfill many requirements for inclusion, while many conditions existed that excluded patients from a diagnosis. Research criteria, therefore, have a high specificity by design and, consequently, a low sensitivity. The definition of research criteria by the NIDDK can be considered to have been a milestone in the facilitation of research of IC. The NIDDK criteria have been widely used ever since, not only for research but also in clinical settings.

11.2 Where Were We off Base?

Despite the fact that the NIDDK criteria were never intended for the diagnosis of individual patients in clinical practice, they were often used as such. Not surprisingly, they were found to have a low sensitivity: they were fulfilled by only one third of patients thought to have IC by experts [2]. The low sensitivity for the diagnosis of IC had two serious consequences:

1. Many patients who were considered by experts to suffer from IC, did not get this diagnosis (clinical problem). In general, "*no diagnosis*" means "*no treatment*" in clinical practice. Even if treatment is given in this situation, problems may exist with reimbursement by insurance companies.
2. The group of patients with a research diagnosis in no way formed a good representation of the disease in the population (research problem). Results obtained in these selected and non-representative patient groups were often incorrectly extrapolated to all patients with the disease.

11.3 What Seminal Publications Changed Our Thinking?

Three seminal publications changed our thinking on interstitial cystitis. It should be realized, however, that the results of studies of many investigators during the past 30 years paved the way for them. These publications were on standardization [3], diagnosis [4] and glomerulations [5].

J.P. van de Merwe
Erasmus MC, Department of Immunology, Rotterdam, The Netherlands
e-mail: email@jpvandemerwe.nl

P.M. Hanno et al. (eds.), *Bladder Pain Syndrome – An Evolution*,
https://doi.org/10.1007/978-3-319-61449-6_11

11.3.1 Standardization

At a meeting in Kyoto (Japan) in 2003, aimed at producing an acceptable definition of IC, it became clear that the way IC patients were evaluated differed enormously between centres [3]. Substantial differences in the approach to IC were also apparent between Europe and North America. As a specific definition of IC seemed unlikely if patient evaluation is not performed in a standardized way, 23 European physicians interested in IC therefore met in Copenhagen in May 2003 in an attempt to reach a consensus on how to perform the evaluation of patients with suspected IC. The meeting was very fruitful and recommendations for medical history, physical examination, laboratory tests, symptom evaluation, urodynamics, assessment of maximum bladder capacity, cystoscopy (technique, inspection, classification), and morphology (technique and number of biopsies, biopsy handling, mast cell counting) were accepted by all participants [3].

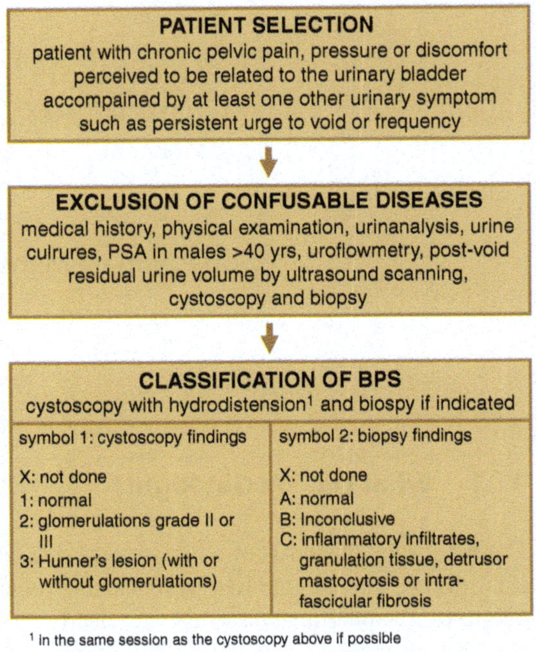

Fig. 11.1 Schematic representation of the proposed steps in the diagnosis of bladder pain syndrome (BPS) including patient selection, exclusion of confusable diseases and classification of BPS

11.3.2 Diagnostic Criteria

At ESSIC meetings in Baden (Austria) in 2005 and in London (United Kingdom) in 2006, the use of separate sets of criteria for clinical diagnoses and research was considered impractical and unwanted. Moreover, criteria should make diagnoses possible in the great majority of—if not all—patients that were considered by experts to have the disease. ESSIC tried to solve these problems by following the way a diagnosis is usually made in clinical practice. This implied the following simplified steps (Fig. 11.1):

1. Definition of patients who should be investigated for interstitial cystitis/bladder pain syndrome (BPS).
2. Definition of diseases with overlapping and/or similar features to BPS, the so-called confusable diseases. This is an important step as many of the confusable diseases can and/or should be treated and/or be cured.
3. Patients in whom a confusable disease is unlikely to be the main cause of the symptoms and/or signs are further investigated for BPS.
4. An important aspect is that all patients who fulfill step 1 are classified on the basis of the findings. To make this possible it became evident that this required definition of types of BPS based on the findings. Disease typing within a diagnosis is not new and has shown to have major advantages in malignancies.

11.3.2.1 Selection of Patients

It was agreed that further investigations for BPS should be done for patients with chronic (>6 months) pelvic pain, pressure, or discomfort perceived to be related to the urinary bladder accompanied by at least one other urinary symptom such as persistent urge to void or increased frequency.

11.3.2.2 Confusable Disease: Diagnosis or Exclusion

Confusable diseases as the cause of the symptoms must be excluded. Table 11.1 shows the diseases that were discussed and accepted as confusable diseases for BPS with an indication as to how they can be recognized or excluded. However, a diagnosis of a confusable disease does not necessarily exclude a diagnosis of BPS. This is relevant for patients in whom treatment of the confusable disease does not resolve their urinary symptoms.

11.3.2.3 Classification of BPS

Consensus was obtained that hydrodistension at cystoscopy was a prerequisite for the documentation of positive but not mandatory signs for the diagnosis of BPS, and if indicated also a

Table 11.1 Confusable diseases for bladder pain syndrome (BPS)

Confusable disease	Excluded or diagnosed by[a]
Carcinoma and carcinoma *in situ*	Cystoscopy and biopsy
Infection with	
Common intestinal bacteria	Routine bacterial culture
Chlamydia trachomatis, Ureaplasma urealyticum,	Special cultures
Mycoplasma hominis, Mycoplasma genitalium,	
Corynebacterium urealyticum, Candida species	
Mycobacterium tuberculosis	Dipstick; if "sterile" pyuria culture for *M. tuberculosis*
Herpes simplex and *Human Papilloma Virus*	Physical examination
Radiation	Medical history
Chemotherapy, including immunotherapy with cyclophosphamide	Medical history
Anti-inflammatory therapy with tiaprofenic acid	Medical history
Bladder neck obstruction and neurogenic outlet obstruction	Uroflowmetry and ultrasound
Bladder stone	Imaging or cystoscopy
Lower ureteric stone	Medical history and/or haematuria: upper urinary tract imaging such CT or IVP
Urethral diverticulum	Medical history and physical examination
Urogenital prolapse	Medical history and physical examination
Endometriosis	Medical history and physical examination
Vaginal candidiasis	Medical history and physical examination
Cervical, uterine and ovarian cancer	Physical examination
Incomplete bladder emptying (retention)	Post-void residual urine volume measured by ultrasound scanning
Overactive bladder	Medical history and urodynamics
Prostate cancer	Physical examination and PSA
Benign prostatic obstruction	Uroflowmetry and pressure-flow studies
Chronic bacterial prostatitis	Medical history, physical examination, culture
Chronic non-bacterial prostatitis	Medical history, physical examination, culture
Pudendal nerve entrapment	Medical history, physical examination, nerve block may prove diagnosis
Pelvic floor muscle related pain	Medical history, physical examination

CT computed tomography, *IVP* intravenous pyelogram, *PSA* prostate-specific antigen
[a]The diagnosis of a confusable disease does not necessarily exclude a diagnosis of BPS

Table 11.2 Classification of types of bladder pain syndrome on the basis of findings at cystoscopy with hydrodistension and of biopsies

Cystoscopy with hydrodistension					
		Not done	Normal	Glomerulations[a]	Hunner's lesion[b]
Biopsy	Not done	XX	1X	2X	3X
	Normal	XA	1A	2A	3A
	Inconclusive	XB	1B	2B	3B
	Positive[c]	XC	1C	2C	3C

[a]Cystoscopy: glomerulations grade 2–3
[b]With or without glomerulations
[c]Histology showing inflammatory infiltrates and/or detrusor mastocytosis and/or granulation tissue and/or intrafascicular fibrosis

biopsy to document histologic details of BPS [4]. Cystoscopic features that were accepted as positive signs of BPS were glomerulations grade 2–3 or Hunner lesions, or both. Histologic findings that were accepted as positive signs of BPS were inflammatory infiltrates and/or granulation tissue and/or detrusor mastocytosis and/or intrafascicular fibrosis.Table 11.2 shows the proposed classification of types of BPS on the basis of findings at cystoscopy with hydrodistension and of biopsies. It is likely that BPS types in individual patients may change over time.

11.3.2.4 Hunner Lesion

ESSIC realized that despite its name, Hunner's ulcer is not a chronic ulcer but rather a distinctive inflammatory lesion presenting a characteristic deep rupture through the mucosa and submucosa provoked by bladder distension. The word ulcer suggests incorrectly that it can always be seen at cystoscopy without hydrodistension. Consequently, ESSIC proposed to replace the name Hunner's ulcer by Hunner lesion. The following definition by M. Fall was accepted: "The Hunner lesion typically presents as a circumscript, reddened mucosal area with small vessels radiating towards a central scar, with a fibrin deposit or coagulum attached to this area. This site ruptures with increasing bladder distension, with petechial oozing of blood from the lesion and the mucosal margins in a waterfall manner. A rather typical, slightly bullous edema develops post-distension with varying peripheral extension" [4].

11.4 Glomerulations

Recently, a systematic literature search showed no consistent relationship between glomerulations and the diagnosis of bladder pain syndrome/interstitial cystitis [5]. It also became evident that there were many contradictory results between the studies. Evidence was found that the grade of glomerulations changed with time. No link was found between the severity of symptoms and the number of glomerulations. There were studies that found glomerulations in healthy asymptomatic populations as well as in symptomatic populations with another primary diagnosis. One study showed no glomerulations in an asymptomatic population. The results of the review are in line with previous considerations on glomerulations [6].

11.5 Where Do We Go from Here?

11.5.1 Glomerulations and the Diagnosis of BPS

The recent conclusions from the systematic literature review on glomerulations [5] raises the question as to whether the finding of grade 2–3 glomerulations should be removed from the ESSIC criteria for the diagnosis of BPS. Common sense suggests that they should be removed and the only consequence would be that glomerulations would be considered to be a normal finding and that all BPS types 2 will become BPS types 1.

In general, symptoms and signs for use in diagnostic criteria do not need to be specific for the disease in question. On the contrary, if a specific symptom or sign existed for the disease, a diagnosis would only require the presence of the specific feature and diagnostic criteria would not be necessary [7].

From a scientific viewpoint, however, there are severe objections to removal of them from the criteria at this stage. The reason is that the reviewed studies on glomerulations were not designed to answer the question as to whether or not glomerulations should have a place in diagnostic criteria. Consequently, the review does not allow conclusions on the value of glomerulations in the ESSIC criteria. Moreover, there is no world-wide consensus on the significance of glomerulations for the diagnosis and prognosis of BPS/IC. The ESSIC criteria for the diagnosis of BPS are an excellent tool to answer the question on the value of glomerulations for the diagnosis and prognosis of BPS types in future studies. Removal of glomerulations from the criteria would make this almost impossible.

11.5.1.1 BPS Type 3C

BPS type 3C is identical to what used to be called interstitial cystitis with Hunner's ulcer or Hunner's type. Several investigators suggest to remove BPS type 3C from the current ESSIC BPS types and consider it as a separate disease with the preferred name of interstitial cystitis. There are several arguments against such a change at this stage. Previously ESSIC reached consensus on changing the name of interstitial cystitis into bladder pain syndrome (BPS) because the name BPS was in line with the other chronic pelvic pain syndromes and was in balance with the clinical presentation of the syndrome and the level of knowledge of its pathophysiology [4]. Moreover, the name interstitial cystitis had become meaningless because of the complete lack of a working definition. Knowledge concerning the etiology and pathophysiology has not significantly changed over the last 10 years for any of the BPS types. Nevertheless, it is evident that patients with BPS type 3C represent a more homogeneous and better defined patient group than any of the other BPS types. It is likely that such a group probably gives a better possibility to detect etiologic and/or pathogenic mechanisms.The ESSIC criteria for the diagnosis of BPS are an excellent tool to answer the question as to whether BPS type 3C is different disease to other BPS types once new findings on the cause of BPS become apparent.

11.5.1.2 Course of BPS

Little is known on the natural course of the various BPS types. It is not known whether BPS type 3C is preceded by any of the other types or *vice versa*. Such studies would be prone to biases by the fact that Hunner lesions may go undetected when cystoscopy is performed without hydrodistension.

In addition, little is known regarding the response to treatment and prognosis for different BPS types. Here too, the ESSIC criteria for the diagnosis of BPS are an excellent tool to answer questions as to whether there is a relationship between BPS types and clinical course, response to treatment and prognosis.

References

1. Gillenwater JY, Wein AJ. Summary of the National Institute of Arthritis, Diabetes, Digestive and Kidney Diseases Workshop on Interstitial Cystitis, National Institutes of Health, Bethesda, Maryland, August 28-29, 1987. J Urol. 1988;140:203–6.
2. Hanno PM, Landis JR, Matthews-Cook Y, Kusek J, Nyberg L Jr. The diagnosis of interstitial cystitis revisited: lessons learned from the National Institutes of Health Interstitial Cystitis Database study. J Urol. 1999;161:553–7.
3. Nordling J, Anjum FH, Bade JJ, Bouchelouche K, Bouchelouche P, Cervigni M, Elneil S, Fall M, Hald T, Hanus T, et al. Primary evaluation of patients suspected of having interstitial cystitis (IC). Eur Urol. 2004;45:662–9.
4. van de Merwe JP, Nordling J, Bouchelouche P, Bouchelouche K, Cervigni M, Daha LK, Elneil S, Fall M, Hohlbrugger G, Irwin P, et al. Diagnostic criteria, classification, and nomenclature for painful bladder syndrome/interstitial cystitis: an ESSIC proposal. Eur Urol. 2008;53:60–7.
5. Wennevik GE, Meijlink JM, Hanno P, Nordling J. Glomerulations in bladder pain syndrome: a review. J Urol. 2016;195:19–25.
6. Sant G. Diagnosis of interstitial cystitis: a clinical, endoscopic and pathologic approach. In: Hanno PM,

Staskin DR, Krane RJ, Wein AJ, editors. Interstitial cystitis. London: Springer; 1990. p. 107–14.
7. van de Merwe JP, Nordling J, Bouchelouche P, Cervigni M, Fall M, Wyndaele J-J. Diagnostic criteria, classification, and nomenclature for bladder pain syndrome (BPS). In: Nordling J, Wyndaele J-J, van de Merwe JP, Bouchelouche P, Cervigni M, Fall M, editors. Bladder pain syndrome: a guide for clinicians. New York: Springer; 2013. p. 21–33.

12 Diagnosis of Interstitial Cystitis: A Comment on Glomerulations

Gjertrud Egge Wennevik

12.1 What Did We Get Right?

Thirty years ago Sant recognized that glomerulations were not pathognomonic for BPS. And it was recognized that glomerulations were present in many other conditions such as radiation cystitis and carcinoma in situ. This is still true today. And studies published in recent years showed that glomerulations also appear in a range of other conditions, such as upper urinary tract stones, BPH/LUTS and prostatitis, as well as in asymptomatic populations [1–6].

Sant also argues that cystoscopic findings frequently do not correlate with symptoms or response to treatment. This stance has not been challenged in the last 30 years when considering glomerulations. Recent studies have not shown any link between severity of symptoms and the grade of glomerulations [7–10].

Cystoscopy should still be a prerequisite for establishing the diagnosis of BPS, as the diagnosis of carcinoma in situ, and other confusable diseases as recommended by the ESSIC consensus should be ruled out before making the diagnosis.

G.E. Wennevik
Department of Urology, Zealand University Hospital, Roskilde, Denmark
e-mail: gjertrud.w@gmail.com

12.2 Where Were We Off Base?

Glomerulations, although present in many patients with BPS, is not considered a hallmark of BPS syndrome anymore [11]. Countless studies have demonstrated the presence of glomerulations in patients without symptoms of BPS, and they cannot be linked to severity of symptoms or bladder capacity under anesthesia. Also some studies suggest that up to 35% of a population with BPS did not have glomerulations [12, 13]. These studies indicate that the occurrence of glomerulations no longer have any value in clinical diagnostics of BPS [11].

12.3 Which Seminal Publications Changed Our Thinking?

Waxman et al. 1998 published the first double blinded study where the occurrence of glomerulations was studied in an asymptomatic population [1]. This study found the prevalence to be as high in the symptomatic group as in the asymptomatic. Although this study was published in 1998, there has been no repeat blinded study looking for glomerulations in asymptomatic populations, but in later years several studies have been published that show glomerulations in patients with other urological conditions, such as BPH/LUTS. Another important study was conducted by Wyndaele et al., who found that 24% of patients with severe BPS symptoms had no glo-

P.M. Hanno et al. (eds.), *Bladder Pain Syndrome – An Evolution*,
https://doi.org/10.1007/978-3-319-61449-6_12

merulations [10]. Also Simon et al., and Richter et al. showed that the occurrence of glomerulations in patients with BPS vary greatly [12, 13].

Recently a large number of studies were summarized in an in-depth review by Wennevik et al. The authors of this review suggested that glomerulations are not related specifically to BPS, nor are they useful clinically in diagnosis, prognosis, or selection of therapy.

12.4 Where Do We Go from Here?

Glomerulations as we understand them now have no clinical significance, and should not be used diagnostically or for phenotyping. Further research should be conducted to investigate if glomerulations have any significance in ways we do not fully understand today. Perhaps they are involved in pathophysiology in some patients? We can conclude however that glomerulations should not be used clinically before we have more insight.

References

1. Waxman JA, Sulak PJ, Kuehl TJ. Cystoscopic findings consistent with interstitial cystitis in normal women undergoing tubal ligation. J Urol. 1998;160:1663.
2. Berger RE, Miller JE, Rothman I, et al. Bladder petechiae after cystoscopy and hydrodistension in men diagnosed with prostate pain. J Urol. 1998;159:83.
3. Furuya R, Masumori N, Furuya S, et al. Glomerulation observed during transurethral resection of the prostate for patients with lower urinary tract symptoms suggestive of benign prostatic hyperplasia is a common finding but no predictor of clinical outcome. Urology. 2007;70:922.
4. Hassan AA, Elgamal SA, Sabaa MA, et al. Evaluation of intravesical potassium sensitivity test and bladder biopsy in patients with chronic prostatitis/chronic pelvic pain syndrome. Int J Urol. 2007;14:738.
5. Jiang, Y.-H., Lee, C.-L., Jhang, J.-F. et al.: 1143 Development of Bladder Glomerulations After Hydrodistension in Patients With Upper Urinary Tract Urolithiasis Suggesting Cross Talk and Bladder Inflammation Occur Between Upper and Lower Urinary Tract. The Journal of Urology, 189: e466.
6. Chung MK, Butrick CW, Chung CW. The overlap of interstitial cystitis/painful bladder syndrome and overactive bladder. JSLS. 2010;14:83.
7. Messing E, Pauk D, Schaeffer A, et al. Associations among cystoscopic findings and symptoms and physical examination findings in women enrolled in the Interstitial Cystitis Data Base (ICDB) Study. Urology. 1997;49:81.
8. Cole EE, Scarpero HM, Dmochowski RR. Are patient symptoms predictive of the diagnostic and/or therapeutic value of hydrodistention? Neurourol Urodyn. 2005;24:638.
9. Ottem DP, Teichman JM. What is the value of cystoscopy with hydrodistension for interstitial cystitis? Urology. 2005;66:494.
10. Wyndaele JJ, Van Dyck J, Toussaint N. Cystoscopy and bladder biopsies in patients with bladder pain syndrome carried out following ESSIC guidelines. Scand J Urol Nephrol. 2009;43:471.
11. Wennevik GE, Meijlink JM, Hanno P, et al. The role of glomerulations in bladder pain syndrome: a review. J Urol. 2016;195:19.
12. Richter B, Hesse U, Hansen AB, et al. Bladder pain syndrome/interstitial cystitis in a Danish population: a study using the 2008 criteria of the European Society for the Study of Interstitial Cystitis. BJU Int. 2010;105:660.
13. Simon LJ, Landis JR, Erickson DR, et al. The interstitial cystitis data base study: concepts and preliminary baseline descriptive statistics. Urology. 1997;49:64.

Diagnosis of Interstitial Cystitis

13

Jörgen Quaghebeur

The term 'interstitial cystitis' has been replaced by BPS introducing a new nomenclature, based on diagnostic and classification criteria [1, 2].

The etiology of IC/BPS is poorly understood, and its pathogenesis may involve multiple pathways leading to a common clinical entity [3].

Frequency, urgency and pain on bladder filling are the most common symptoms of BPS. All urodynamic volumes are reduced. Associated conditions include psychological distress, depression, history of sexual assault, irritable bowel syndrome and fibromyalgia. Cystoscopy remains the test for definitive diagnosis, with visualization of hemorrhage on cystoreduction. A multidisciplinary treatment approach is essential in the management of this condition [4]. An association between anxiety disorder (AD) and IC/BPS has been shown. Clinicians should evaluate and monitor the presence of IC/BPS in patients with AD [5]. Sexual dysfunction was an important component of IC/BPS phenotype, and adding a sexual dysfunction domain to the UPOINT system improved the association with IC/BPS symptom severity [6].

No structural ANS abnormalities in IC/BPS subjects have been shown. Higher baseline heart rate (HR) supports the concept of functional rather than structural change in the ANS, such as abnormality of sympathetic/parasympathetic balance that will require further evaluation [7]. Altered sensory processing in patients with IC/BPS may result from a deficiency of the central nervous system to adequately filter incoming visceral afferent information [8]. White matter abnormalities closely correlated with symptoms of IC/BPS, including bladder pain and urinary symptoms. These anatomical brain alterations suggest that there are neuropathological contributions to chronic urological pelvic pain [9]. Changes in somatosensory gray matter may have an important role in pain sensitivity as well as affective and sensory aspects of interstitial cystitis [10]. Women with IC/BPS have a sensorimotor component to the pathological condition involving an alteration in intrinsic oscillations and connectivity in a cortico-cerebellar network previously associated with bladder function [11].

The classic type of interstitial cystitis with Hunner's lesions, bladder pain syndrome type 3C according to current terminology, stands out as a well-defined phenotype; it has to be evaluated separately in clinical studies and practice, as treatment requirements differ importantly between this and other phenotypes [12].

Publications did not indicate specific questionnaires able to show symptom differences between type 3C and non-type 3C BPS. Literature presents no questionnaires able to differentiate subtypes of BPS (e.g. type 3C and non-type 3C

J. Quaghebeur
Department of Urology, University Hospital Antwerp, Wilrijkstraat 10, Edegem B 2650, Belgium
e-mail: jorgen.quaghebeur@telenet.be

P.M. Hanno et al. (eds.), *Bladder Pain Syndrome – An Evolution*,
https://doi.org/10.1007/978-3-319-61449-6_13

BPS). We suggest using the ESSIC guideline to differentiate between subgroups in BPS [13, 14].

A thorough clinical assessment including a 'four step protocol' for investigation of CPPS has been proposed, aiming to obtain supplementary information to refine the therapeutic management. The 'four step protocol' involves: (step 1) a careful history with questioning for complaints in other systems. The evaluation of previous assessments and reports (step 2). Step 3 involves an extensive clinical assessment (e.g. neurological, hernia's (e.g. inguinal, Spighelian), an assessment the external sex organs and the small pelvis via rectal and vaginal ways). The extensive clinical assessment of the musculoskeletal system (step 4) includes an assessment of the full spine and pelvic girdle. Muscular pain, tendons and pain points have to be determined. Attention for emotional consequences as a result of the chronic suffering is important assessing patients with CPPS [14–17].

Analysis of multiple urinary proteins and serum cytokines could provide a diagnostic basis for IC/BPS, and could be a tool for the differential diagnosis of IC/BPS and other sensory bladder disorders [18]. Urodynamic tests, cystoscopy and hydrodistension, biopsies and pathologic evaluation are in the process of finding a place in the diagnostic tree [19]. Correlations between cystoscopic findings, maximal bladder capacity and bladder histology were found [20]. Over active bladder (OAB) and IC/BPS are different symptoms complexes that share urgency as a common symptom. None of them have a specific symptom although pain on bladder filling is the hallmark symptom in IC/BPS [21]. There is considerable overlap of self-reported symptoms between IC/BPS and OAB. This overlap raises the possibility that the two conditions represent a continuum of a bladder hypersensitivity syndrome [22].

Analysis of multiple urinary proteins and serum cytokines could provide a diagnostic basis for IC/BPS, and could be a tool for the differential diagnosis of IC/BPS and other sensory bladder disorders [18, 23, 24]. Urinary nerve growth factor (NGF) but not prostaglandin E2 increases in patients with IC/BPS and detrusor overactivity [25]. There is an increased level of NGF in the IC/BPS patients [26].

One of the most common findings in IC bladders is denudation or thinning of the bladder epithelium, suggesting an altered regulation of urothelial homeostasis [27]. Glomerulations should be included in the diagnosis or phenotyping of IC/BPS. Glomerulations do not correlate with symptoms and are found in patients without IC/BPS [28]. Sensory hyperinnervation and basal urothelial p75NTR staining together with assessment of inflammatory lymphocytes and urothelial integrity allow the differentiation of IC/BPS and overactive bladder syndrome, even in the absence of Hunner lesions. Furthermore, these histopathological criteria enable the identification of early disease stages or oligo-/a-symptomatic cases, and may permit timely treatment to prevent disease progress [29].

Mast cell counting should be done in a standardized way and the pathology report should include several data as proposed before [19]. Twenty seven mast cells/mm^2 is considered indicative of mastocytosis [30]. Mast cell density does not appear to correlate with duration of symptom amelioration after complete transurethral resection of Hunner's lesions [31]. Subepithelial mast cell distribution was characteristic of IC/BPS with Hunner lesions. Detrusor mastocytosis had poor predictive value for IC/BPS. Mast cell assessment did not distinguish IC/BPS without Hunner lesions from overactive bladder syndrome [32].

References

1. Nordling J, Wyndaele JJ, van de Merwe JP, Bouchelouche P, Cervigni M, Fall M, editors. Bladder pain syndrome: a guide for clinicians. New York: Springer; 2013. p. 389.
2. van de Merwe JP, Nordling J, Bouchelouche P, Bouchelouche K, Cervigni M, Daha LK, Elneil S, Fall M, Hohlbrugger G, Irwin P, Mortensen S, van Ophoven A, Osborne JL, Peeker R, Richter B, Riedl C, Sairanen J, Tinzl M, Wyndaele JJ. Diagnostic criteria, classification, and nomenclature for painful bladder syndrome/interstitial cystitis: an ESSIC proposal. Eur Urol. 2008;53:60–7.
3. Arora HC, Shoskes DA. The enigma of men with interstitial cystitis/bladder pain syndrome. Transl Androl Urol. 2015;4:668–76.
4. Offiah I, McMahon SB, O'Reilly BA. Interstitial cystitis/bladder pain syndrome: diagnosis and management. Int Urogynecol J. 2013;24:1243–56.

5. Chung KH, Liu SP, Lin HC, Chung SD. Bladder pain syndrome/interstitial cystitis is associated with anxiety disorder. Neurourol Urodyn. 2014;33:101–5.
6. Liu B, Su M, Zhan H, Yang F, Li W, Zhou X. Adding a sexual dysfunction domain to UPOINT system improves association with symptoms in women with interstitial cystitis and bladder pain syndrome. Urol. 2014;84:1308–13.
7. Chelimsky G, McCabe NP, Janata J, Elston R, Zhang L, Ialacci S, Chelimsky T. Autonomic testing of women with interstitial cystitis/bladder pain syndrome. Clin Auton Res. 2014;24:161–6.
8. Kilpatrick LA, Ornitz E, Ibrahimovic H, Hubbard CS, Rodriguez LV, Mayer EA, Naliboff BD. Gating of sensory information differs in patients with interstitial cystitis/painful bladder syndrome. J Urol. 2010;184:958–63.
9. Farmer MA, Huang L, Martucci K, Yang CC, Maravilla KR, Harris RE, Clauw DJ, Mackey S, Ellingson BM, Mayer EA, Schaeffer AJ, Apkarian AV. Brain white matter abnormalities in female interstitial cystitis/bladder pain syndrome: a MAPP Network Neuroimaging Study. J Urol. 2015;194:118–26.
10. Kairys AE, Schmidt-Wilcke T, Puiu T, Ichesco E, Labus JS, Martucci K, Farmer MA, Ness TJ, Deutsch G, Mayer EA, Mackey S, Apkarian AV, Maravilla K, Clauw DJ, Harris RE. Increased brain gray matter in the primary somatosensory cortex is associated with increased pain and mood disturbance in patients with interstitial cystitis/painful bladder syndrome. J Urol. 2015;193:131–7.
11. Kilpatrick LA, Kutch JJ, Tillisch K, Naliboff BD, Labus JS, Jiang Z, Farmer MA, Apkarian AV, Mackey S, Martucci KT, Clauw DJ, Harris RE, Deutsch G, Ness TJ, Yang CC, Maravilla K, Mullins C, Mayer EA. Alterations in resting state oscillations and connectivity in sensory and motor networks in women with interstitial cystitis/painful bladder syndrome. J Urol. 2014;192:947–55.
12. Fall M, Logadottir Y, Peeker R. Interstitial cystitis is bladder pain syndrome with Hunner's lesion. Int J Urol. 2014;21:79–82.
13. Quaghebeur J, Wyndaele JJ. Bladder pain syndrome (BPS): symptom differences between type 3C BPS and non-type 3C BPS. Scand J Urol. 2015;49:319–20.
14. Quaghebeur J, Wyndaele JJ. A review of techniques used for evaluating lower urinary tract symptoms and the level of quality of life in patients with chronic pelvic pain syndrome. Itch Pain. 2015;2:e659.
15. Fall M. The complexity of chronic pelvic pain. In: Defoe® editor, ESSIC, 2015 Abstract book International Society for the Study of interstitial cystitis/bladder pain syndrome. Italy; 2015. p. 3–4.
16. Quaghebeur J. Research on diagnostic techniques used in CPPS patients. Wilrijk, Faculty of Medicine and Health Sciences. Doctor in Medical Sciences, Antwerp University; 2015. p. 149.
17. Quaghebeur J, Wyndaele JJ. Chronic pelvic pain syndrome: role of a thorough clinical assessment. Scand J Urol. 2015;49:81–9.
18. Kuo HC. Potential urine and serum biomarkers for patients with bladder pain syndrome/interstitial cystitis. Int J Urol. 2014;21:34–41.
19. Wyndaele JJ. Evaluation of patients with painful bladder syndrome/interstitial cystitis. Scientific World J. 2005;5:942–9.
20. Wyndaele JJ, Van Dyck J, Toussaint N. Cystoscopy and bladder biopsies in patients with bladder pain syndrome carried out following ESSIC guidelines. Scand J Urol Nephrol. 2009;43:471–5.
21. Castro-Diaz D, Cardozo L, Chapple CR, Espuna M, Kelleher C, Kirby M, Milsom I, Sievert KD, Tubaro A. Urgency and pain in patients with overactive bladder and bladder pain syndrome. What are the differences? Int J Clin Pract. 2014;68:356–62.
22. Lai HH, Vetter J, Jain S, RWt G, Andriole GL. The overlap and distinction of self-reported symptoms between interstitial cystitis/bladder pain syndrome and overactive bladder: a questionnaire based analysis. J Urol. 2014;192:1679–85.
23. Hanno P. Editorial comment from Dr Hanno to potential urine and serum biomarkers for patients with bladder pain syndrome/interstitial cystitis. Int J Urol. 2014;21:41.
24. Yoshimura N. Editorial comment from Dr Yoshimura to potential urine and serum biomarkers for patients with bladder pain syndrome/interstitial cystitis. Int J Urol. 2014;21:42.
25. Liu HT, Tyagi P, Chancellor MB, Kuo HC. Urinary nerve growth factor but not prostaglandin E2 increases in patients with interstitial cystitis/bladder pain syndrome and detrusor overactivity. BJU Int. 2010;106:1681–5.
26. Chen W, Ye DY, Han DJ, GQ F, Zeng X, Lin W, Liang Y. Elevated level of nerve growth factor in the bladder pain syndrome/interstitial cystitis: a meta-analysis. Spring. 2016;5:1072.
27. Ke QS, Kuo HC. Pathophysiology of interstitial cystitis/bladder pain syndrome. Tzu Chi Medical Journal. 2015;27:139–44.
28. Wennevik GE, Meijlink JM, Hanno P, Nordling J. The role of glomerulations in bladder pain syndrome: a review. J Urol. 2016;195:19–25.
29. Regauer S, Gamper M, Fehr MK, Viereck V. Sensory hyperinnervation distinguishes bladder pain syndrome/interstitial cystitis from overactive bladder syndrome. J Urol. 2016;197:159–66.
30. Larsen MS, Mortensen S, Nordling J, Horn T. Quantifying mast cells in bladder pain syndrome by immunohistochemical analysis. BJU Int. 2008;102: 204–7. discussion 7
31. Rössberger J, Fall M, Gustafsson CK, Peeker R. Does mast cell density predict the outcome after transurethral resection of Hunner's lesions in patients with type 3C bladder pain syndrome/interstitial cystitis? Scand J Urol Nephrol. 2010;44:433–7.
32. Gamper M, Regauer S, Welter J, Eberhard J, Viereck V. Are mast cells still good biomarkers for bladder pain syndrome/interstitial cystitis? J Urol. 2015;193:1994–2000.

14 Commentary on Sant Chapter: 30 Years on!

Grannum R. Sant

14.1 30-Year Historical Overview of Interstitial Cystitis (IC)

2017 is the 30th anniversary of the First NIH-NIDDK Conference on Interstitial Cystitis that was held in at the NIH in Bethesda, Maryland, USA in August 1987. It is thus an appropriate and opportune time to review progress made over the last three decades in the understanding of this still enigmatic disease and to highlight progress in understanding the disease pathophysiology, epidemiology, diagnosis and treatment.

Prior to the August 1987 NIH Workshop on IC, there was scant attention paid in medical and urological circles to IC with the generally held view that IC was a "psychosomatic disease". This nihilistic diagnostic and therapeutic consensus only began to change with the formation of the Interstitial Cystitis Association (ICA) by Vicki Ratner MD in 1984. The first urology journal Supplement exclusively devoted to IC was published in April 1987 [1] 4 months before the landmark NIH Workshop that defined IC for "research studies" [2].

The number of publications on IC has increased exponentially since the watershed year of 1987—first Journal Supplement and NIH Workshop. PubMed publications in the 5-year period 1982–1987 were 181 increasing to 314 between 1988–1993 and 1129 in the most recent 5-year period.

Since 1987 millions of dollars have been committed by the NIH-NIDDK to fund studies of IC and many pharmaceutical and biotechnology companies have endeavoured to develop innovative treatments for patients suffering from IC. Disappointingly, in spite of the government, industry and foundation funding and the explosion of publications no new IC treatment has achieved FDA regulatory approval in the United States (US) since Elmiron (pentosan polysulfate sodium) in 1996–21 years ago (see Table 14.1). The only other treatment for IC approved in the USA is intravesical dimethyl sulfoxide (DMSO) approved in 1978—the year that the non-ulcer form of IC was described by Messing and Stamey from Stanford University.

Table 14.1 Abbreviated IC timelines summary

• 1978 Non-ulcer IC described
• 1984 Formation of Interstitial Cystitis Association (ICA) patient advocacy group
• 1987 First urology Journal Supplement devote to IC
• 1990 First Conference Proceedings book on IC (Springer–Verlag)
• 1997 First IC textbook (Lippincott)
• FDA drug approvals
– Intravesical DMSO 1978
– Oral Pentosanpolysulfate (Elmiron) 1996

G.R. Sant, M.D., F.R.C.S., F.A.C.S.
Emeritus Professor and former Chairman of the Department of Urology, Tufts University School of Medicine, Boston, MA 02111, USA
e-mail: grannum.sant@yahoo.com

P.M. Hanno et al. (eds.), *Bladder Pain Syndrome – An Evolution*,
https://doi.org/10.1007/978-3-319-61449-6_14

14.2 What We Got Right?

Despite the current demonstrable unmet medical patient need for new therapies there are many issues that the field got right. IC is no longer regarded as an orphan disease as it was in 1987 and multiple studies have shown that it is not uncommon in men—frequently misdiagnosed as prostatodynia and/or non-bacterial prostatitis.

The global awareness of the disease has improved significantly with ongoing research and patient education activities extending from the US to Europe, South America, Asia- Pacific, India and South Africa. There have been special journal issues on IC published with the most recent the October and December issues of Translational Andrology and Urology (TAU) in 2015.

14.3 What We Got Wrong?

In 1987 the majority opinion among urologists was that diagnosis required a cystoscopy under anesthesia ("glomerulations", Hunner's ulcers) and biopsy showing pathologic inflammation ("cystitis") of the bladder wall. Currently IC is a diagnosis of exclusion of known bladder diseases (bacterial infection, cancer, carcinoma-in-situ) and based on a symptom complex similar to that of the overactive bladder syndrome (OAB). Recently the distinction between ulcer (Hunner) and non-ulcer forms of the disease have gained some cachet as it may well be that both forms have distinct pathophysiology and treatments?

The diagnostic criteria for research studies of IC defined at the 1987 NIH Workshop [2] has been confined to the dustbin of history and has been replaced by a symptom-based definition and exclusion of known bladder disease.

Another paradigm shift from 30 years ago has to do with pathophysiology and disease progression—namely, is IC a primary bladder disease or a pelvic floor disease? Originally it was thought that IC starts in the bladder (altered bladder wall permeability) leading to bladder wall inflammation ("interstitial cystitis") and subsequent up-regulation of the sensory nerves in the sub-urothelium, pelvic floor, pelvic organs (bowel, female genital organs) and lower spinal cord. Current thoughts on pathobiology focus on IC as a component of a pelvic pain syndrome and hence the additional definitions of Bladder Pain Syndrome (BPS), Painful Bladder Syndrome (PBS) and Hypersensitive Bladder (HSB) [3].

14.4 What's in a Name—Nomenclature "Redux"?

IC has been defined and redefined by multiple regional organizations (US, Europe, Asia Pacific) and no consensus terminology has emerged. The confusing stew of definitions—Interstitial Cystitis (IC), Painful Bladder Syndrome (PBS), Bladder Pain Syndrome (BPS) and Hypersensitive Bladder (HSB) has resulted in a lack of uniformity of disease definition and a degree of confusion for clinicians, researchers, patients and reimbursement authorities.

This definitional "over-reach" is regrettable and confusing for patients, reimbursement entities, epidemiologists and healthcare systems (see Table 14.2).

Not all IC patients have bladder or pelvic pain although they complain of urgency and suprapubic discomfort. In my clinical experience about one third of IC patients do not have pain. This begs the question as to the use of pain (in Bladder Pain Syndrome) and painful (as in Painful Bladder Syndrome) in the various names/definitions of interstitial cystitis. Is it time for all global organizations and societies to come together and agree upon a simple and unified definition of IC?

Table 14.2 A personal wish list for the next 5–10 years

• Definitional parsimony with a single disease name
• Increased human studies (symptoms, tissue etc.)
• Application of new genomic/precision medicine tools
• Better understanding of disease pathophysiology
• Is IC a primary bladder or pelvic disease?
• Is ulcer IC different from non-ulcer IC?
• Regulatory approval of new oral/intravesical therapies

The relationship of IC to OAB needs clarification. Is IC a pain subset of OAB or can IC be categorized into two subsets—with and without pelvic pain? Hopefully the NIH-NIDDK MAPP research network can clarify and categorize IC subsets.

A review of the 30-year history of the Interstitial Cystitis Association (ICA) patient advocacy group highlights lessons learnt regarding the value of advocacy groups to patients, clinicians, researchers and funding agencies. The confusing proliferation of disease definitions for IC is cogently articulated and effectively challenged by the founder of the International Painful Bladder Foundation (IPBF) [3]. Hopefully her recent plea for a "patient-centered" standardization does not fall on deaf ears!

Awareness of the disease has increased as a result of the sterling work and contribution of various patient advocacy groups in public education and political lobbying and the increased funding of IC research worldwide. Sadly the large amount of basic science and other research, mainly funded by the National Institutes of Health (NIH-NIDDK) has not translated into any new FDA drug approval since 1996 when sodium pentosanpolysulfate was approved based on its Phase 3 registration study [4].

My personal IC wish list for the next 5–10 years is tablulated in Table 14.2.

14.5 Important Publications in Last 30 Years—Personal Selection

Since the NIH-NIDDK Workshop on IC in the summer of 1987 there has been an explosion of interest and scientific/medical publications on the disease Interstitial Cystitis (IC).

Following is a brief summary of important publications in the last 30 years. Since the publication of the first textbook on IC in 1997 [5], there has been no further editions, updates or other textbooks. This is a void that needs filling.

The validation of the O'Leary-Sant questionnaire [6] resulted in near universal acceptance of this patient reported outcomes measure as a quantifiable endpoint in clinical studies of IC.

Interstitial cystitis in men has been repeatedly described and most men with non-bacterial prostatitis/prostatodynia are now felt to be suffering from IC [7].

The 2012 randomized trial of myofascial physical therapy [8] cemented the place of this treatment modality in the therapeutic armamentarium and supported the thinking that IC/BPS was a pelvic rather than a primary bladder disease.

The American Urological Association guidelines publication on diagnosis and treatment of IC/BPS was widely acclaimed both upon its initial publication and recent update in 2015 [9].

A multi-disciplinary approach to diagnosis and treatment of IC is now standard in many IC clinics and referral centers worldwide. The Beaumont Hospital group in Michigan, USA has been one of the original proponents of this holistic approach [10].

14.6 Summary and Conclusions

The last 30 years of research and increased awareness of the disease has resulted in only one drug approval in the USA in 1996. This is disappointing especially from the patient and patient advocacy perspectives. Researchers, funders, clinicians and patients need to come together to reset the research agenda and speed up the research ecosystem for moving from basic science to translational research and transfer into the clinic. The long-suffering IC patient deserves no less in 2017.

References

1. Sant GR, editor. Interstitial cystitis-1987. Urology. 1987;25(4):1–48.
2. Gillenwater JY, Wein AJ. Summary of the National Institute of Arthritis, Diabetes, Digestive and Kidney Diseases Workshop on Interstitial Cystitis, National Institutes of Health, Bethesda, Maryland, August 28–29, 1987. J Urol. 1988;140(1):203–6.

3. Meijlink JM. Patient-centered standardization in interstitial cystitis/bladder pain syndrome-a PLEA. Transl Androl Urol. 2015;4(5):499–505.
4. Parsons CL, Benson G, Childs SJ, Hanno P, Sant GR, Webster G. A quantitatively controlled method to study prospectively interstitial cystitis and demonstrate the efficacy of Pentosanpolysulfate. J Urol. 1993;150(3):845–8.
5. Sant GR, editor. Interstitial cystitis. Philadelphia: Lippincott–Raven Press; 1997.
6. Lubeck DP, Whitmore K, Sant GR, Alvarez-Horine S, Lai C. Psychometric validation of the O'Leary-Sant interstitial cystitis symptom index in a clinical trial of pentosan polysulfate sodium. Urology. 2001;57(6 Suppl 1):62–6.
7. Forrest JB, Nickel JC, Moldwin RM. Chronic prostatitis/chronic pelvic pain syndrome and male interstitial cystitis: enigmas and opportunities. Urology. 2007;69(4 Suppl):60–3.
8. FitzGerald MP, Payne CK, Lukacz ES, Yang CC, Peters KM, Chai TC, Nickel JC, Hanno PM, Kreder KJ, Burks DA, Mayer R, Kotarinos R, Fortman C, Allen TM, Fraser L, Mason-Cover M, Furey C, Odabachian L, Sanfield A, Chu J, Huestis K, Tata GE, Dugan N, Sheth H, Bewyer K, Anaeme A, Newton K, Featherstone W, Halle-Podell R, Cen L, Landis JR, Propert KJ, Foster HE Jr, Kusek JW, Nyberg LM, Interstitial Cystitis Collaborative Research Network. Randomized multicenter clinical trial of myofascial physical therapy in women with interstitial cystitis/painful bladder syndrome and pelvic floor tenderness. J Urol. 2012;187(6):2113–8.
9. Gupta P, Gaines N, Sirls LT, Peters KM. A multidisciplinary approach to the evaluation and management of interstitial cystitis/bladder pain syndrome: an ideal model of care. Transl Androl Urol. 2015;4(6):611–9.
10. Hanno PM, Erickson D, Moldwin R, Faraday MM. Diagnosis and treatment of interstitial cystitis/bladder pain syndrome: AUA guideline amendment. J Urol. 2015;193(5):1545–53.

15 Neuro-Urologic Evaluation in Interstitial Cystitis

Jean Jacques Wyndaele

There has been quiet an evolution about knowledge of BPS since Ed McGuire wrote this chapter.

The terminology has changed, the value of different tests has become clearer. The international understanding of BPS as "symptom syndrome" and not "disease" has opened new perspectives, and created new challenges.

As BPS is a syndrome with symptoms found in many different conditions, a stepwise diagnosis is needed, which starts with the clinical possibility that the patient suffers from BPS, the performance of consequent tests to exclude confusable diseases, putting all data together in order to define which type of BPS pathology is present and leading to the best decision for what should be the primary treatment, and eventually further steps.

It is a fact that pain is the major symptom. Sensation is subjective, and pain sensation per definition will show very different levels and localisations depending on the individual. Is it nociceptive pain or rather neuropathy? Its subjectivity does not mean that symptom reporting is unreliable or not valid. It is the main thing available to indicate that there is a pain causing condition in the pelvic region. Problematic may be that tests can grade and better define the pain but not prove that pain actually exists.

J.J. Wyndaele
Department of Urology, Antwerp University, GGW, Wilrijk, Antwerp, Belgium
e-mail: wyndaelejj@skynet.be

15.1 What Did We Get Right?

Neuro-urological diagnostic techniques have so far fairly little to offer in the investigation of BPS patients, beside for excluding other conditions.

That differential diagnosis with Overactive Bladder can be important in patients complaining of urgency and frequency, and discomfort is correct.

It has been shown that hyperactivity of the striated pelvic muscles/urethral sphincter is present in many BPS patients. It remains uncertain if this is cause, consequence or both.

That BPS patients mostly show discomfort when the bladder is filled to smaller than considered normal volumes is correct. But not in all patients such a relation can be seen. Though several pathophysiological mechanisms have been hypothesized the exact cause of this increased sensation remains uncertain.

It is likely that different types of sensory innervation play and that sensory information which leads to bladder contraction is different from the pain related mechanisms.

The limited role of urodynamic tests is accepted by many, though considered important in the differential diagnosis with OAB.

Patients with BPS but with normal bladder capacity under anaesthesia are not rare. There is no evidence that the cases with general macroscopic pathology of the bladder wall or with Hunner lesion relate to different neurologic dysfunctions. It needs to be better studied if patients with

P.M. Hanno et al. (eds.), *Bladder Pain Syndrome – An Evolution*,
https://doi.org/10.1007/978-3-319-61449-6_15

different diagnostic findings need to be treated differently. That treatment does anything more than influence the symptomatic expression of the disease rather than cure the condition is likely. If spontaneous cure may happen is uncertain.

15.2 Where Were We off Base?

The neuro-urologic evaluation as described highlights some important reflexions, but focus, based on the knowledge at that time, was somewhat missing. Since publication quite a lot of new knowledge has been acquired.

The terminology "sensory urgency "and "motor urgency "has been abandoned. The latest terminology reports [1, 2] describe genitourinary pain syndromes as constellations, or varying combinations of symptoms, which cannot be used for precise diagnosis.

All bladder pain syndromes are chronic in their nature. Pain is the major complaint but concomitant complaints are of LUT, bowel, sexual or gynecological nature. The suprapubic pain may be related to bladder filling, accompanied by other symptoms such as increased daytime and night-time frequency, in the absence of proven urinary infection or other obvious pathology.

The knowledge on the innervation related to BPS in primary order, second order, third order neurons and in the brain has been extensively described [3]. The different stages in development of the pain: local >peripheral > central > cerebral, known for a long time in other pain conditions [4] are present also in BPS. The importance of making an early diagnosis follows from this, as well as the need to study the influence of duration of the disease on different treatment success. Combination treatments for peripheral and central can be worthwhile [5].

An oversimplified view on the different neurogenic structures involved in BPS pain is not valid anymore. Several things can be mentioned: myelinated mechanoreceptive fibers in the bladder wall also possess chemoreceptive properties [6]; mechanoinsensitive C fibers may become mechanosensitive during inflammation, probably providing a substrate for hypersensitivity (pain, urgency) at lower bladder content [7]. The innervation related to signaling pain from the pelvic region runs not only in the pelvic plexus, but also in the hypogastric nerves [8]. It need to be explored if such animal findings are also happening in humans with BPS. The effects of intravesical vanilloids, and of oxybutinin give credit to this hypothesis [9, 10]. It needs to be developed further how the increased knowledge in basic findings can help improving the phenotyping and choice of treatment modalities.

Best ways to diagnose have been looked at in International Guidelines (as AUA, mentioned here). "Recommended are a basic assessment including a careful history, physical examination, and laboratory examination in order to rule in symptoms that characterize IC/BPS and rule out other confusable disorders. Baseline voiding symptoms and pain levels should be obtained in order to measure subsequent treatment effects. Cystoscopy and/or urodynamics should be considered as an aid to diagnosis only for complex presentations".

ESSIC has developed clear guidelines [11] which have been validated by several groups [12, 13].

Beside the reporting of symptoms by the patients, Questionnaires are frequently used to make data more uniform and make evaluation of the impact of symptoms on quality of life more clear. By filling out most used questionnaires (Mc Gill PQ, MPQ-DLV, PDI, NIH-CPS, ICSI and PUF a wide variety of symptoms and a negative impact of quality of life were found [14]. Both genders had the same lower urinary tract symptoms. Women were less sexually active and had a significantly higher negative impact on the level of quality of life. But when comparing the most used questionnaires, very different results can be found. This indicates that data from one questionnaire cannot be used for overall conclusions concerning pain intensity and QoL. For bladder symptoms, the results seem to correspond better [15]. A literature review did not indicate specific questionnaires able to show symptom differences between cases with or without Hunner lesion [16].

The role of a thorough clinical assessment is high. The "four step plan "stresses the importance to pay also special attention to the musculoskeletal system. It is not difficult to perform and provides valuable information on possible muscular problems and neuropathy [17].

The role of physical examination is mostly to exclude confusable diseases. Sensation of touch in the perineal area is normal unless a very extended sensitization has occurred. Lumbosacral reflexes are normal.

15.3 What Seminal Publications Changed Our Thinking?

- Wyndaele JJ, Malaguti S. Neurophysiology of pelvic pain mechanisms. In: Nordling J, Wyndaele JJ, van de Merwe JP, Bouchelouche P, Cervigni M, Fall M, editors. Bladder pain syndrome. Chapter 6. New York: Springer; 2013. p. 87–102.
- Quaghebeur J, Wyndaele JJ. Prevalence of lower urinary tract symptoms and level of quality of life in men and women with chronic pelvic pain. Scand J Urol. 2015;49:242–249.
- Quaghebeur J, Wyndaele JJ. Comparison of questionnaires used for the evaluation of patients with chronic pelvic pain. Neurourol Urodyn. 2013; 32:1074–1079.
- Quaghebeur J, Wyndaele JJ. Bladder pain syndrome (BPS): Symptom differences between type 3C BPS and non-type 3C BPS. Letter to the editor. Scand J Urol. 2014; 49(4): 319–320.
- Quaghebeur J, Wyndaele JJ. Chronic pelvic pain syndrome: role of a throrough clinical assessment.

15.4 Where Do We Go from Here?

There is need to improve the diagnostic testing in order to permit better phenotyping and as such better guidance to the best available treatment in the single patient.

To develop one generally accepted questionnaire would facilitate the interpretation and comparison of data in this condition.

If overactivity of the pelvic floor/urethral sphincter is cause or consequence or both needs to be studied further.

Whether peripheral neuropathy is more common than currently thought needs to be studied in more detail, as well as the consequences for treatment. Differentiating from e.g. pudendal nerve neuropathy is mandatory.

One cannot stress enough the importance of accurate diagnostic exclusion of other pathologies before definitely accepting the diagnosis of BPS. The danger to use only noninvasive tests have been clearly shown [18] but seems still to be overlooked. Reinvestigation must be considered when little result comes from treatment [19].

References

1. Abrams P, Cardozo L, Fall M, et al. The standardisation of terminology of lower urinary tract function: report from the Standardisation Sub-committee of the International Continence Society. Am J Obstet Gynecol. 2002;187:116–26. Neurourol Urodyn 2002;21:167–178.
2. Haylen BT, de Ridder D, Freeman RM, et al. An International Urogynecological Association (IUGA)/International Continence Society (ICS) joint report on the terminology for female pelvic floor dysfunction. Int Urogynecol J. 2010;21:5–26. Neurourol Urodyn 2010;29:4–20.
3. Wyndaele JJ, Malaguti S. Neurophysiology of pelvic pain mechanisms. In: Nordling J, Wyndaele JJ, van de Merwe JP, Bouchelouche P, Cervigni M, Fall MB, editors. Ladder pain syndrome. Chapter 6. New York: Springer; 2013. p. 87–102.
4. Besson JM. Pain. The neurobiology of pain. Lancet. 1999;353:1610–5.
5. van Ophoven A. From end-organ disease to a classifiable bladder pain syndrome: paradigm shift in the understanding of urological pain syndromes exemplified by the condition currently called interstitial cystitis. Urologe A. 2009;48:156–62.
6. Habler HJ, Janig W, Koltzenburg M. Activation of unmyelinated afferent fibers by mechanical stimuli and inflammation of the urinary bladder in the cat. J Physiol. 1990;425:545–62.
7. Janig W, Koltzenburg M. On the function of spinal primary afferent fibres supplying colon and urinary bladder. J Auton Nerv Syst. 1990;30:S89–96.
8. Moss NG, Harrington WW, Tucker S. Pressure, volume, and chemosensitivity in afferent innervation of urinary bladder in rats. Am J Phys. 1997;272:R695–703.
9. Lazzeri M, Beneforti P, Spinelli M, et al. Intravesical resinefertotoxin fort he treatment of hypersensitive

disorder: a randomized placebo controlled study. J Urol. 2000;164:676–9.
10. Barbalias GA, Liatsikos EN, Athanasopoulos A, et al. Interstitial cystitis: bladder training with intravesical oxybutinin. J Urol. 2000;163:1818–22.
11. van de Merwe JP, Nordling J, Bouchelouche P, et al. Diagnostic criteria, classification, and nomenclature for painful bladder syndrome/interstitial cystitis: an ESSIC proposal. Eur Urol. 2008;53:60–7.
12. Mouracade P, Lang H, Jacqmin D, et al. Using the intersitital cystitis new diagnostic criteria in daily practice: about 156 patients. Prog Urol. 2008;18:674–7.
13. Richter B, Hesse U, Hansen AB, et al. Bladder pain syndrome/interstitial cystitis in a Danish population: a study using the 2008 criteria of the European Society for the Study of Interstitial Cystitis. BJU Int. 2010;105:660–7.
14. Quaghebeur J, Wyndaele JJ. Prevalence of lower urinary tract symptoms and level of quality of life in men and women with chronic pelvic pain. Scand J Urol. 2015;49:242–9.
15. Quaghebeur J, Wyndaele JJ. Comparison of questionnaires used for the evaluation of patients with chronic pelvic pain. Neurourol Urodyn. 2013;32:1074–9.
16. Quaghebeur J, Wyndaele JJ. Bladder pain syndrome (BPS): symptom differences between type 3C BPS and non-type 3C BPS. Letter to the editor. Scand J Urol. 2014;49(4):319–20.
17. Quaghebeur J, Wyndaele JJ. Chronic pelvic pain syndrome: role of a thorough clinical assessment. Scand J Urol. 2015;49(2):81–9.
18. Tissot WD, Diokno AC, Peters KM. A referral center's experince with transitional cell carcinoma misdiagnosed as interstitial cystitis. J Urol. 2004;172:478–80.
19. Irwin P, Samsudin A. Reinvestigation of patients with a diagnosis of interstitial cystitis: common things are sometimes common. J Urol. 2005;174:584–7.

16 Current Role of Neurourologic Evaluation in Interstitial Cystitis/Bladder Pain Syndrome

Hann-Chorng Kuo

In the chapter of neurourologic evaluation in interstitial cystitis (IC) [1], McGuire pointed out that urodynamic study cannot provide strong information as the first step in diagnosis of IC. The role of urodynamic study in the diagnosis of IC is still controversial over 30 years later. In order to identify the small voided volume and frequent urination in BPS patients, a voiding diary has been suggested by Payne to replace urodynamic study [2]. The reason for this is that cystometric bladder capacity may be misleading due to psychological embarrassment and the invasive nature of the procedure. The voiding diary can reflect the true frequency episodes and functional bladder capacity and painful conditions. However, patients might not able to differentiate urgency sensation due to bladder discomfort between BPS and overactive bladder (OAB). The cardinal symptom of BPS is caused by small functional bladder capacity; therefore, one might speculate that urodynamic study might provide additional information to confirm the diagnosis and make treatment strategy decisions [3].

16.1 Terminology: IC, Bladder Pain Syndrome, or Hypersensitive Bladder?

McGuire had stated in his chapter that "sensory urgency is the common urodynamic finding in this discomfort bladder disease." Indeed, IC is characterized by bladder pain, frequency and nocturia. NIDDK broadened the diagnostic criteria of IC and included persistent urge to void or frequency [4]. Although urgency has been a complaint of most patients, the content of urgency complained of by BPS patients is quite different from that which occurs in patients with OAB [5]. In order to solve the confused terminology of IC, the hypersensitive bladder syndrome (with or without pain) has been proposed by Homma Y. [6]. The fundamental diagnostic criteria for IC are bladder pain, reduced bladder capacity, and exclusion of other detectable diseases [4]. Although urodynamic study seems able to identify IC patients with increased bladder sensation and reduced bladder capacity, these urodynamic findings are not pathognomonic signs for IC. In

H.-C. Kuo
Department of Urology, Buddhist Tzu Chi General Hospital, Tzu Chi University, Hualien, Taiwan
e-mail: hck@tzuchi.com.tw

P.M. Hanno et al. (eds.), *Bladder Pain Syndrome – An Evolution*,
https://doi.org/10.1007/978-3-319-61449-6_16

order to increase the diagnostic accuracy, adding potassium sensitivity test (PST) might be helpful [7]. Even though, overlap of IC and OAB diagnosis remains in glomerulations and PST [8].

16.2 What Is the Real Pathophysiology of IC?

It is possible that mild degrees of urothelial dysfunction can also be found in other urinary tract diseases such as urolithiasis, bladder outlet obstruction, and overactive bladder syndrome [9]. These diseases cause urothelial dysfunction and, therefore, patients also have bladder irritative symptoms. If we classify IC according to symptoms and duration, these patients might also be categorized into having IC unless they were excluded by identifying characteristic pathologies. In addition, patients with IC have been found to have higher risks of irritable bowel syndrome, fibromyalgia, general fatigue and functional somatic syndrome, suggesting IC is involved in systemic inflammatory disorders [10–12]. Fluctuation of IC symptoms in non-ulcer IC might result from altered inert immunity from time to time. On the contrary, ulcer type IC might be organ confined disease that is resulted from localized bladder inflammation due to previous insult or trauma. The different IC phenotype and etiologies of disease make these two IC subtypes have different treatment strategy and outcome [13].

McGuire mentioned that some patients with IC might progress to a poorly compliant bladder in association with painful sensation. Urodynamic study provides evidence for an uncontrollable diseased bladder indicating that partial or total cystectomy with augmentation cystoplasty or urinary diversion are necessary. He also mentioned the urethral sphincter hyperactivity in IC. Because urethral striated sphincter activity is associated with inhibition of detrusor contractility, patients with IC usually complain of difficult urinating or interruption of urination. In AUA, EAU, Asian and ICI guidelines on IC, urodynamic study is considered as an optional procedure primarily to exclude other LUTD that might account for the similar IC symptoms [14–17]. However, patients with IC have been found to have increased bladder sensation, reduced bladder capacity, and increased outlet resistance. Some studies have reported a high percentage of IC patients have bladder outlet obstruction [18]. Increase of bladder afferent activities due to chronic inflammation might enhance urethral sphincter tonicity resulting in poor relaxation of pelvic floor muscle during voiding [19]. Whether the presence of bladder outlet obstruction is the cause or effect in the IC patient needs further evaluation. Based on the NIDDK criteria, those patients proven to have bladder outlet obstruction should be excluded from the diagnosis of IC [4]. Clinical research showed significant association between urodynamic variables and the degree of glomerulations after cystoscopic hydrodistention and the severity of clinical symptoms measured by IC symptom index and IC problem index [20].

16.3 Inflammation and Urothelial Dysfunction in IC/BPS

In the original 1990 chapter, McGuire stated "we have not unreasonably assumed that inflammation may be the etiology of the uncomfortable symptoms in patients with interstitial cystitis. However, there is no real proof for that concept, and the actual cause of the uncomfortable bladder symptoms in IC remains unknown". Up to now, IC remains a mysterious bladder disease. IC has been considered as an organ confined (bladder) inflammatory disease, but nowadays it is regarded as a heterogeneous syndrome. Patients might have different etiologies which result in similar clinical symptoms. Urothelial dysfunction, chronic bladder inflammation, and systemic functional disorders have been found closely related to the pathogenesis of IC and bladder pain syndrome (BPS). A distinct phenotype of IC patients with multiple sensitivities is identified

[21]. Recent research on urine and serum biomarkers, and bladder tissue histopathology have also provided evidence for the clinical characteristics of IC, such as urothelial barrier defects, activation of sensory fibers and epitheliolymphocytic infiltration, all of which might contribute to the development of IC [22–25]. However, we still cannot classify IC into different subtypes for appropriate treatment.

Recent research on bladder mucosa have demonstrated that it has not only a barrier function, but also transmits sensory signals [26]. Abnormal urothelial function results in bladder hypersensitivity due to activation of sensory fibers. Abnormal proliferation of urothelial cells leads to immature intermediate cell location in the apical position, which lack barrier function. Inadequate e-cadherin and zonula occludens-1 cause tight junction defects and easy influx of urinary solutes such as potassium [27]. These pathogeneses are believed to result from chronic inflammation in the suburothelium. Increased plasma-lymphocytic cell infiltration has been demonstrated in IC patients with Hunner lesion, in which intense bladder pain and severe frequency urgency are the main symptoms [28].

PST has been recommended to detect the urothelial leakage in patients with IC [7]. However, urothelial leak is not only found in IC bladders but also in the bladders with urothelial cancer, irradiation cystitis, bladder outlet obstruction, overactive bladder or other LUTD [9]. Urothelial leakage is a pathology caused by acute or chronic inflammation in the bladder wall, therefore, any bladder insult that results in urothelial barrier defect may have a positive PST. More severe urothelial dysfunction is more susceptible to the stimulation of potassium, thus resulting in volume reduction in IC patients [20]. A previous study further found that in patients with storage symptoms refractory to medical treatment, small cystometric bladder capacity and a positive PST causing pain and elevated visual analog score, IC is highly likely [29]. The sensitivity of a positive PST in IC patients is higher than the glomerulations after hydrodistention [30].

16.4 Where Is the Role of Urodynamic Test for IC/BPS?

A urodynamic study might not be an essential test for the diagnosis of IC, however, it remains important for (1) the exclusion of bladder outlet obstruction and detrusor overactivity; (2) confirmation of the clinical symptoms of IC; (3) obtaining objective findings of bladder hypersensitivity; (4) determination of bladder compliance; (5) assessing the severity of bladder pathology; and (6) providing objective information when assessing the treatment outcome. Although the value of urodynamic test in the diagnosis of IC/BPS remains inconclusive, the parameters of urodynamic test are associated with IC symptoms, severity of glomerulations and maximal bladder capacity. Urodynamic study reflects the bladder sensory and motor conditions and can exclude other lower urinary tract diseases that have similar IC symptoms. Although not pathognomonic for IC, this objective investigation still provides valuable information in clinical management of IC.

References

1. McGuire E. Neurourologic evaluation in interstitial cystitis. In: Hanno PM, Staskin DR, Krane RJ, Wein AJ, editors. Interstitial cystitis. London: Springer; 1990. p. 114–9.
2. Payne C. Urodynamics for the evaluation of painful bladder syndrome/interstitial cystitis. J Urol. 2010;184: 15–7.
3. Kim SH, Kim TB, Kim SW, Oh SJ. Urodynamic findings of the painful bladder syndrome/interstitial cystitis: a comparison with idiopathic overactive bladder. J Urol. 2009;181:2550–4.
4. National Institute of Diabetes and Digestive and Kidney Diseases: Consenss Meeting on IC/BPS, February 10, 2007. Washington, DC: US Government Printing Office 2007; NIH Publication No. 7–5512.
5. Diggs C, Meyer WA, Langenberg P, Greenberg P, Horne L, et al. Assessing urgency in interstitial cystitis/ painful bladder syndrome. Urology. 2007;69:210–4.
6. Homma Y. Hypersensitive bladder: a solution to confused terminology and ignorance concerning interstitial cystitis. Int J Urol. 2014;21(Suppl 1):43–7.

7. Parsons CL. The role of a leaky epithelium and potassium in the generation of bladder symptoms in interstitial cystitis/overactive bladder, urethral syndrome, prostatitis and gynaecological chronic pelvic pain. BJU Int. 2011;107:370–5.
8. Chung MK, Butrick CW, Chung CW. The overlap of interstitial cystitis/painful bladder syndrome and overactive bladder. JSLS. 2010;14:83–90.
9. Liu HT, Jiang YH, Kuo HC. Alteration of urothelial inflammation, apoptosis, and junction protein in patients with various bladder conditions and storage bladder symptoms suggest common pathway involved in underlying pathophysiology. Low Urin Tract Symptoms. 2015;7:102–7.
10. Martinez-Martinez LA, Mora T, Vargas A, Fuentes-Iniestra M, Martinez-Lavin M. Sympathetic nervous system dysfunction in fibromyalgia, chronic fatigue syndrome, irritable bowel syndrome, and interstitial cystitis: a review of case-control studies. J Clin Rheumatol. 2014;20:146–50.
11. Warren JW, Morozov V, Howard FM, et al. Before the onset of interstitial cystitis/bladder pain syndrome, the presence of multiple non-bladder syndromes is strongly associated with a history of multiple surgeries. J Psychosom Res. 2014;76:75–9.
12. Nickel JC, Tripp DA, International Interstitial cystitis study Group. Clinical and psychological parameters associated with pain pattern phenotypes in women with interstitial cystitis/bladder pain syndrome. J Urol. 2015;193:138–44.
13. Offiah L, McMahon SB, O'Reilly BA. Interstitial cystitis/bladder pain syndrome: diagnosis and management. Int Urogynecol J. 2013;24:1243–56.
14. Hanno PM, Buks DA, Clemens JQ, Dmochowski RR, Erickson D, et al. AUA guideline for the diagnosis and treatment of interstitial cystitis/bladder pain syndrome. J Urol. 2011;185:2162–70.
15. Merwe JPVD, Nordling J, Bouchelouche P, Bouchelouche K, Cervigni M, et al. Diagnostic criteria, classification, and nomenclature for painful bladder syndrome/interstitial cystitis: an ESSIC proposal. Eur Urol. 2008;53:60–7.
16. Hanno P, Lin A, Nordling J, Nyberg L, Ophoven AV, et al. Bladder pain syndrome international consultation on incontinence. Neurol Urodynam. 2010;29:191–8.
17. Homma Y, Ueda T, Tomoe H, Lin ATL, Kuo HC, et al. Clinical guidelines for interstitial cystitis and hypersensitive bladder syndrome. Int J Urol. 2009;16:597–615.
18. Cameron AP, Gajewski JB. Bladder outlet obstruction in painful bladder syndrome/interstitial cystitis. Neurourol Urodyn. 2009;28:944–8.
19. McGuire EJ, Shin-Chun Z, Horwinski ER, Lytton B. Treatment of motor and sensory instability by electrical stimulation. J Urol. 1983;129:775–8.
20. Kuo YC, Kuo HC. The urodynamic characteristics and prognostic factors of patients with interstitial cystitis/bladder pain syndrome. Int J Clin Pract. 2013;67:863–9.
21. Fuoco MB, Irvine-Bird K, Curtis NJ. Multiple sensitivity phenotype in interstitial cystitis/bladder pain syndrome. Can Urol Assoc J. 2014;8:E758–61.
22. Hauser PJ, Dozmorov MG, Bane BL, Slobodov G, Culkin DJ, Hurst RE. Abnormal expression of differentiation related proteins and proteoglycan core proteins in the urothelium of patients with interstitial cystitis. J Urol. 2008;179:764–9.
23. Zhang CO, Wang JY, Koch KR, Keay S. Regulation of tight junction proteins and bladder epithelial paracellular permeability by an antiproliferative factor from patients with interstitial cystitis. J Urol. 2005;174:2382–7.
24. Keay S, Kaczmarek P, Zhang CO, et al. Normalization of proliferation and tight junction formation in bladder epithelial cells from patients with interstitial cystitis/painful bladder syndrome by d-proline and d-pipecolic acid derivatives of antiproliferative factor. Chem Biol Drug Des. 2011;77:421–30.
25. Homma Y, Nomiya A, Tagaya M, et al. Increased mRNA expression of genes involved in pronociceptive inflammatory reactions in bladder tissue of interstitial cystitis. J Urol. 2013;190:1925–31.
26. Lori B, de Groat WC. Mechanism of disease: involvement of the urothelium in bladder dysfunction. Nat Clin Pract Urol. 2007;4:46–54.
27. Shie JH, Kuo HC. Higher levels of cell apoptosis and abnormal E-cadherin expression in the urothelium are associated with inflammation in patients with interstitial cystitis/painful bladder syndrome. BJU Int. 2011;108:E136–41.
28. Maeda D, Akiyama Y, Morikawa T, Kunita A, Ota Y, et al. Hunner-type (classic) interstitial cystitis: a distinct inflammatory disorder characterized by pancystitis, with frequent expansion of clonal B-cells and epithelial denudation. PLoS One. 2015;20:e0143316.
29. Kuo YC, Kuo HC. Potential factors that can be used to differentiate between interstitial cystitis/painful bladder syndrome and bladder oversensitivity in women. Int J Clin Pact. 2011;66:146–51.
30. Jiang YH, Jhang JF, Kuo HC. Revisiting the role of potassium sensitivity testing and cystoscopic hydrodistention for the diagnosis of interstitial cystitis. PLoS One. 2016;11(3):e0151692. doi:10.1371/journal.pone.0151692.

17 Neurourological Evaluation in BPS

Arndt van Ophoven

Together with Helmuth Madersbacher and others Ed McGuire is one of the most prominent promotors of urodynamic studies in Urology and has thus become a doyen of modern Neuro-Urology. In summary, the entire Chap. 11 by McGuire deals with the potential and limitations of urodynamics as a diagnostic tool to identify BPS/IC or to at least distinguish it from confusable disorders. The introductory statement by McGuire is still valid 30 years later, i.e. that urodynamics cannot provide the definite diagnosis of BPS/IC.

Whatever you prefer to call it, whatever sophisticated connotation or attribution you will add to your preferred definition or classification of this condition, first and foremost BPS/IC is a pain syndrome, a health constraint basically due to pain. Thus, the statement that "neurourological techniques have little to offer as a *first step* in the investigation of patients with this kind of symptomology" appears to be still correct and true. Moreover, patients are typically unhappy to undergo urodynamic testing, not infrequently complaining about discomfort and pain, sometimes resulting in anxiety [3, 6]. This is particularly true for patients with complaints of chronic pelvic pain syndromes.

A. van Ophoven, M.D., Ph.D.
Division of Neuro-Urology, Marien Hospital Herne, University Hospital Ruhr-Universität Bochum, Hölkeskampring 40, 44625 Herne, Germany
e-mail: arndt.vanophoven@marienhospital-herne.de

McGuire's historical wording, e.g. *sensory and motor urgency* has been superceded (at least for now) and has been substituted by alternative taxonomy and classifications regarding urodynamic recordings and findings. However, the fact that urodynamics have remained a challenging tool to decipher BPS/IC has not changed. Urodynamics are still under debate for the work up of BPS/IC patients and are, in contrast to some guidelines and recommendations, not unanimously performed in daily practice for this purpose [2, 4].

The thoughtful discussion by Payne and Blaivas on pros and cons of urodynamics for the evaluation of patients presenting with BPS/IC cannot substantially be nourished or further elaborated [1, 5]. To my personal point of view each physician is currently left to his/her own decision as to at what point the patient should undergo urodynamic testing, basically to expand the input of diagnostic information while striving for optimized management of BPS/IC patients.

References

1. Sastry DN, Hunter KM, Whitmore KE. Urodynamic testing and interstitial cystitis/painful bladder syndrome. Int Urogynecol J. 2010;21(2):157–61.
2. Kim SH, Kim TB, Kim SW, Oh SJ. Urodynamic findings of the painful bladder syndrome/interstitial cystitis: a comparison with idiopathic overactive bladder. J Urol. 2009;181(6):2550–4.

P.M. Hanno et al. (eds.), *Bladder Pain Syndrome – An Evolution*,
https://doi.org/10.1007/978-3-319-61449-6_17

3. Solomon ER, Ridgeway B. Interventions to decrease pain and anxiety in patients undergoing urodynamic testing: a randomized controlled trial. Neurourol Urodyn. 2016;35(8):975–9.
4. Payne C. Urodynamics for the evaluation of painful bladder syndrome/interstitial cystitis. J Urol. 2010;184(1):15–6.
5. Blaivas JG. Urodynamics for the evaluation of painful bladder syndrome/interstitial cystitis. J Urol. 2010;184(1):16–7.
6. Yeung JY, Eschenbacher MA, Pauls RN. Pain and embarrassment associated with urodynamic testing in women. Int Urogynecol J. 2014;25(5):645–50.

Bladder Hydrodistension in 2017

18

Claus Riedl

The role of bladder hydrodistension as an important diagnostic and therapeutic tool in bladder pain syndrome/interstitial cystitis (BPS/IC), as popularized by Messing and Stamey in 1978, has been significantly questioned within the last years. For many decades the "disease-specific" glomerulations, petechial mucosal bleedings, have been regarded to be pathognomonic for BPS/IC and, thus, included in the National Institute of Diabetes and Digestive and Kidney Diseases (NIDDK) criteria to better define patients suffering from this disease [1]. As a proposed scale for disease severity, glomerulations have even been graded with regard to their extension and intensity [2].

A recent review of publications on glomerulations in BPS/IC showed no consistent relationship between glomerulations and the diagnosis of BPS/IC. Several studies were not able to demonstrate a link between symptom severity and the number of glomerulations. Some investigators also observed that the grade of glomerulations may change with time. Glomerulations were observed in healthy asymptomatic populations as well as in symptomatic populations with another primary diagnosis. In summary, the authors found no convincing evidence that glomerulations should be included in the diagnosis or phenotyping of BPS/IC [3].

The fact that hydrodistension gives temporary symptom relief to a considerable number of BPS/IC patients was first reported by Bumpus in 1930 [4] and made it one of the few available therapeutic regimens for many years. Even in 2017, the mechanism for this symptom remission is not understood. Partial sensory denervation of suburothelial nerve plexus by hydrodistension pressure is one of the presumed mechanisms for symptom remission, and axonal degeneration has been observed in animal studies after bladder overdistension [5]. Chai found a significant increase of urinary heparin-binding epidermal growth factor (HB-EGF) and a significant decrease of urinary anti-proliferative factor (APF) after in vivo bladder stretch [6]. Bägli described an increased expression of RHAMM (receptor for hyaluronic acid mediated motility) after bladder stretch, which may be an early step for tissue repair in response to injured bladder tissue [7]. Within the last 15 years, no more studies on the physiologic effects of bladder hydrodistension have been published, and only two publications from this period refer to the clinical outcome of this procedure:

Glemain reported on the results of 32 BPS/IC patients that were treated prospectively by continuous balloon dilatation of the bladder for 3 h under epidural anesthesia. The intravesical pressure used was equal to the patients mean arterial pressure. Pain resolution was maintained for

C. Riedl
Department of Urology, Landesklinikum Baden-Moedling, Waltersdorfer Str. 75, 2500 Baden, Austria
e-mail: claus.riedl@baden.lknoe.at

P.M. Hanno et al. (eds.), *Bladder Pain Syndrome – An Evolution*,
https://doi.org/10.1007/978-3-319-61449-6_18

6 months in 60% of patients, and for 1 year in 43.3%. Results were better for patients with a cystometric bladder capacity ≥150 cc before treatment [8].

Hoke treated 106 BPS/IC patients with bladder hydrodistension, of whom 48 simultaneously received a transvaginal trigonal block with 0.25% bupivacaine/1% lidocaine under cystoscopic guidance. Patients with and without trigonal block perceived a significant improvement in pain scores, with no difference between both groups. Distension times of 2 and >5 min did not give statistically different results [9].

A recent publication followed patients after a combination of hydrodistension and fulguration of Hunner's ulcers. The mean time to therapeutic failure (defined as restart with any disease-specific therapy) was 28.5 months in Hunner type and 25.2 months in non-Hunner type disease, with no significant difference for both types of disease [10]. However, it is not clear which procedure was responsible for this long-term symptom improvement and if the combination was necessary to achieve these good results.

Sequential therapy with hydrodistension and intravesical instillation of hyaluronic acid under general anesthesia was performed by several authors: Ahmad found a 74% response rate in 17 patients [11], and Shao reported on a 77.8% response rate at 6 and a 50% response rate at 9 months (compared to 33.3% and 20% with heparin instillations) [12]. Good immediate response with this regimen was also reported by Yang [13].

No publications exist on the long-term course of patients with repeated bladder hydrodistensions after symptom recurrence. Hydrodistension never cures BPS/IC. Whether repeat fulgurations/resections or bladder distensions add to the disease caused bladder wall fibrosis is not known. It is therefore uncertain if aggressive therapy like fulguration/resection or hydrodistension carries a potential negative effect. Theoretically, repeat fulgurations/resections over many years might result in chronic injury to the bladder wall and lead to bladder fibrosis and shrinkage. Whether such changes reflect merely the natural course of the disease or are augmented by these attempts at therapy is unknown. The fibrotic small capacity bladder is the classical indication for bladder augmentation or urinary diversion. Thus, the price to be paid for temporary symptom improvement could be major surgery at a later phase of life. This is important information for patients who are offered hydrodistension for symptomatic relief, since alternative therapeutic regimens do not bear this theoretical consequence.

With this information, the value of bladder hydrodistension in BPS/IC management will most probably be minimized in the future. In principle, the procedure has been performed with roughly the same standards throughout the last decades. The ESSIC definition from 2008 established a maximum intravesical pressure of 80 cm H_2O for 5 min, and glomerulations observed after hydrodistension were rated grade I to III with regard to their extension [2].

Instead of general or spinal anesthesia, local anesthesia with electromotive administration (EMDA) of intravesical lidocaine may be used for painless hydrodistension of the bladder [14]. Rosamilia reported on 21 women who underwent hydrodistension after EMDA with lidocaine and dexamethasone [15]. A good response was observed in 85% of patients 2 weeks after treatment, with 63% still responding at 2 months. 25% of patients were still free of symptoms at 6 months. The same regimen was used by Riedl in 13 patients, and 62% showed complete symptom resolution after an average 4.5 months [16].

Bladder hydrodistension is not a riskless procedure. In the original textbook chapter by Nehra and Vardi, the incidence of bladder ruptures was 8%. Vesical necrosis following hydrodistension has also been reported [17–19]. These events are severe complications that require major surgery for repair and need to be communicated to patients before the intervention.

18.1 Intraoperative Urodynamics During Hydrodistension

The authors of the orginal textbook chapter, Nehra and Vardi, published the only report on urodynamics in BPS/IC patients under general anesthesia. They hypothesized that they could obtain more information about bladder compliance with this procedure, that has not become a standard in BPS/IC evaluation. However, it may harbor interesting information regarding pathophysiology of disease.

In a series of 20 patients they observed bladder hypersensitivity with a mean maximum awake capacity (immediately before general anesthesia) of 275 mL (45–350), defined as onset of pain, and a normal compliance up to this threshold, while under anesthesia non-compliance of the detrusor was recorded in most cases when this maximum capacity was exceeded.

It is not clear if this information was or is valuable. The range of maximum awake capacity is quite high in this series, and the average of 275 mL does not suggest severe reduction of bladder capacity in most cases.

In cases of non-compliance of the bladder under anesthesia elasticity of the bladder wall is most probably reduced by partial fibrosis. Spasticity of the detrusor does not seem to be an explanation, since muscle fibers should be relaxed in general anesthesia. It has been reported that autonomic responses, i.e.significant increases of systolic/diastolic blood pressure and heart rate, are typically found in patients with visible bladder lesions after hydrodistension, and these were concordant with symptom severity [20, 21].

From personal experience, two observations can be reported:

1. Even under general anesthesia, patients with severe BPS/IC start to react when bladder distension reaches a distinct volume. This may be reflected by the autonomic responses measured by Stav and Kim and the bladder non-compliance observed by Nehra and Vardi.
2. Patients with high-volume bladder capacity and minimal/no glomerulations at hydrodistension are no good candidates for cystectomy and may not be pain-free after major surgery. In these cases, origin of pain seems to be different than the urinary bladder.

In summary, hydrodistension under anesthesia may give temporary symptom relief in BS/IC. Combination with EMDA, hyaluronic acid or fulguration seems to improve response rates. The procedure is minimally invasive and may be repeated at symptom recurrence; no data about effectiveness of repeat treatments exist. However, as with repeated fulgurations or resections, repeated hydrodistension may induce bladder fibrosis and shrinkage and finally lead to cystectomy due to minimal bladder capacity.

18.2 What Did We Get Right?

Bladder hydrodistension has been better positioned in BPS/IC: it does not essentially contribute to diagnosis of BPS/IC and has been included in the treatment guidelines (AUA) only as third-line therapy after non-invasive and possibly more effective behavioral and medical regimens.

18.3 Where Were We Off Base?

Despite our present position, bladder hydrodistension may have assisted in better understanding of BPS/IC by stratification of patients. However, it did not prove well as a diagnostic or therapeutic strategy and was replaced by more sophisticated algorithms regarding disease definition and more disease-specific therapeutic regimens.

18.4 What Seminal Publications Changed Our Thinking?

The publications from the ESSIC group and the AUA guidelines, created after extensive discussion among experts and including their huge experience on BPS/IC.

18.5 Where Do We Go from Here?

While the present criteria seem to almost perfectly define BPS/IC patients and the UPOINT system valuably assists as a diagnostic algorithm with regard to the origin of disease, it is still necessary to find better therapies. Bladder hydrodistension will most probably not be part of it. The big task is early detection of disease, which is still lacking in many parts of the world, even if it is not clear if this helps to prevent disease progression to more severe conditions.

References

1. National Institute of Diabetes and Digestive and Kidney Diseases: Consensus Meeting on IC/BPS, February 10, 2007. Washington, DC: US Government Printing Office 2007; NIH Publication No. 7-5512.
2. Merwe JPVD, Nordling J, Bouchelouche P, Bouchelouche K, Cervigni M, et al. Diagnostic criteria, classification, and nomenclature for painful bladder syndrome/interstitial cystitis: an ESSIC proposal. Eur Urol. 2008;53:60–7.
3. Wennevik GE, Meijlink JM, Hanno P, Nordling J. The role of glomerulations in bladder pain syndrome: a review. J Urol. 2016;195:19–25.
4. Bumpus HC. Interstitial cystitis: its treatment by overdistension of the bladder. Med Clin North Am. 1930;13:1495.
5. Sehn JT. The ultrastructural effect of prolonged distension on the neuromuscular apparatus of the bladder. M.Sc. thesis, University of Oxford, 1976.
6. Chai TC, Zhang CO, Shoenfelt JL, Johnson HW, Warren JW, Keays S. Bladder stretch alters urinary heparin-binding epidermal growth factor and antiproliferative factor in patients with interstitial cystitis. J Urol. 2000;163:1440–4.
7. Bägli DJ, Joyner BD, Mahoney SR, McCulloch L. The hyaluronic acid receptor RHAMM is induced by stretch injury of rat bladder in vivo and influences smooth muscle cell contraction in vitro. J Urol. 1999;162:832–40.
8. Glemain P, Riviére C, Lenormand L, Karam G, Bouchot O, Buzelin JM. Prolonged hydrodistention of the bladder for symptomatic treatment of interstitial cystitis: efficacy at 6 months and 1 year. Eur Urol. 2002;41:79–84.
9. Hoke TP, Goldstein H, Saks EK, Vakili B. Hydrodistention of the bladder for the treatment of bladder pain syndrome/interstitial cystitis (BPS/IC). Neurourol Urodyn. 2017;36(3):784–6. doi:10.1002/nau.23024.
10. Niimi A, Nomiya A, Yamada Y, et al. Hydrodistension with or without fulguration of hunner lesions for interstitial cystitis: long-term outcomes and prognostic predictors. Neurourol Urodyn. 2016;35:965–9.
11. Ahmad I, Sarath Krishna NB, Meddings RN. Sequential hydrodistension and intravesical instillation of hyaluronic acid under general anaesthesia for treatment of refractory interstitial cystitis: a pilot study. Int Urogynecol J Pelvic Floor Dysfunct. 2008;19:543–6.
12. Shao Y, Shen ZJ, Rui WB, Zhou WL. Intravesical instillation of hyaluronic acid prolonged the effect of bladder hydrodistention in patients with severe interstitial cystitis. Urology. 2010;75:547–50.
13. Yang JY, Wei W, Lan YL, Liu JQ, Wang HB, Li S. Role of bladder hydrodistention and intravesical sodium hyaluronate in the treatment of interstitial cystitis. Urol J. 2015;12:2417–21.
14. Gürpinar T, Wong HX, Griffith DP. Electromotive administration of intravesical lidocaine in patients with interstitial cystitis. J Endourol. 1996;10:443–7.
15. Rosamilia A, Dwyer PL, Gibson J. Electromotive drug administration of lidocaine and dexamethasone followed by cystodistension in women with interstitial cystitis. Int Urogynecol J Pelvic Floor Dysfunct. 1997;8:142–5.
16. Riedl CR, Knoll M, Plas E, Pflüger H. Electromotive drug administration and hydrodistention for the treatment of interstitial cystitis. J Endourol. 1998;12:269–72.
17. Platte RO, Parekh M, Minassian VA, Poplawsky D. Spontaneous bladder rupture following cystoscopy with hydrodistention and biopsy in a female patient with interstitial cystitis. Female Pelvic Med Reconstr Surg. 2011;17:149–52.
18. Grossklaus DJ, Franke JJ. Vesical necrosis after hydrodistension of the urinary bladder in a patient with interstitial cystitis. BJU Int. 2000;86:140–1.
19. Zabihi N, Allee T, Maher MG, Mourtzinos A, Raz S, Payne CK, Rodriguez LV. Bladder necrosis following hydrodistention in patients with interstitial cystitis. J Urol. 2007;177:149–52.
20. Stav K, Lang E, Fanus Z, Leibovici D. Autonomic response during bladder hydrodistention in patients with bladder pain syndrome. J Urol. 2012;188:117–21.
21. Kim SW, Son HS, Troya IS, Kim JY, Kim MJ, Fraser MO, Kim JH. Autonomic response during bladder hydrodistention reflects the severity of symptoms in patients with bladder pain syndrome/interstitial cystitis. Neurourol Urodyn. 2016;36(3):677–82. doi:10.1002/nau.22994.

19 Pharmacologic Goals in Interstitial Cystitis/Bladder Pain Syndrome

Antonella Giannantoni, Marilena Gubbiotti, Naoki Yoshimura, and Karl-Erik Andersson

During the last 30 years, a number of treatments and management algorithms have been developed and applied in the treatment of patients with Interstitial Cystitis/Bladder Painful Syndrome (IC/BPS), and many behavioral, dietary, interventional, pharmacologic and surgical therapies have been developed in the attempt to control the disease and to offer substantial benefits to the affected patients. Nevertheless, the complexity of the disease in terms of aetiology and pathogenesis still has made it difficult to induce significant and long-lasting benefits for any kind of these treatments. In addition, few well designed, randomised controlled trials have been conducted until now on different treatment modalities, and this still precludes the development of evidence-based management strategies. Indeed, the majority of pharmacological agents used to treat patients with IC/BPS are still off label. In this respect, the Interstitial Cystitis Data Base study noted >180 treatment modalities for IC/BPS, with poor results in the majority of cases [1]. To date, there is general agreement on the use of some agents, orally or intravesically administered, as indicated by the EAU guidelines on chronic pelvic pain [2] and the AUA Guidelines for the Diagnosis and Treatment of Interstitial Cystitis/ Bladder Pain Syndrome [3].

The actual, general picture about the pharmacological treatment of IC/BPS is different compared to that of 30 years ago, when the first edition of the present book was created. Unfortunately the picture has changed only in terms of the high number of pharmacological agents used along time, but not in terms of evidence-based treatment strategies [4–6]. However, efforts have been made to create symptom-based definitions including ESSIC [2, 7] and AUA [3] guidelines of IC/BPS, which were intended to include the entire spectrum of disorders resulting in bladder pain. These guidelines have been used to search for effective systemic or local pharmacotherapies for this difficult disease; however, most therapies still lack a high level of evidence with few recommended treatment options. This is in part due to inadequate patient selection, resulting in heterogeneity of the treated group [8]. Thus, phenotyping of the disease condition based on symptom classification such as the UPOINT system [9] and/or cystoscopic findings of bladder-specific pathophysiology such as Hunner lesion, which fulfils the requirements for classic IC

A. Giannantoni, M.D., Ph.D. (✉)
M. Gubbiotti, M.D.
Urology Section, Department of Surgical and Biomedical Sciences, University of Perugia, Perugia, Italy
e-mail: antonella.giannantoni@unipg.it

N. Yoshimura, M.D., Ph.D.
Department of Urology, School of Medicine, University of Pittsburgh, Pittsburgh, PA 15213, USA
e-mail: nyos@pitt.edu

K.-E. Andersson, M.D., Ph.D.
Institute for Regenerative Medicine, Wake Forest University School of Medicine, Winston Salem, NC, USA
e-mail: karl-erik.andersson@med.lu.se

P.M. Hanno et al. (eds.), *Bladder Pain Syndrome – An Evolution*,
https://doi.org/10.1007/978-3-319-61449-6_19

[10], is important for the selection of appropriate treatments in individual patients. Almost 50% of patients referred to a tertiary IC/BPS clinic, regardless of the complexity or severity of condition, experienced clinically significant improvement using an individualized phenotype-directed therapeutic approach [9].

19.1 What Did We Get Right?

Several of the therapeutic option available in 1988 are still used and even if their weaknesses were adequately pointed out at that time, the documentation of effect (or lack of it) is still incomplete. Below we will update the currently available pharmacotherapies and look into future potential options based on clinical evidence from IC/BPS clinical trials, with which we could also shed some light on different pathophysiological aspects of the disease.

19.2 Current Therapies

19.2.1 Glycosaminoglycan (GAG)-Like Agents

Disruption of the mucin GAG layer of the bladder urothelium has been implicated in the pathogenesis of IC/BPS. The main components of the GAG layer include chondroitin sulfate, hyaluronic acid (HA), heparin sulfate, dermatan sulfate, and keratin sulfate [11]. Therapeutic GAG or GAG-like agents, such as HA, chondroitin sulfate, heparin, and pentosanpolysulfate have been previously used with variable and somewhat disapponting results [12–14].

Pentosan polysulfate sodium (PPS), a synthetic sulphated polysaccharide, is the most frequently GAG-like agent used to replace defective GAGs. Since the preliminary study of Parsons and coworkers in 1983 [15], this agent has been used orally or intravesically administered, in a number of studies. PPS is the only oral medication for IC/BPS approved by the US Food and Drug Administration. The study with the longest follow-up with oral PPS remains that of Hanno and co-workers [16]. In this study, oral PPS 100 mg three times daily induced about a 50% positive response in pain and urgency in IC/BPS patients. PPS has been used alone or in combination with different pharmacological agents [17–20]. In randomized controlled studies, with different doses of oral PPS for different times, the drug has been compared with placebo, heparin, hydroxyzine, cyclosporine A, intravesical liposomes, intravesical PPS, bladder hydrodistension [14, 21–25].

One double-blind, placebo-controlled trial reported subjective improvement in pain, urgency and frequency in patients taking PPS compared to the control group [23]. Longer durations of treatment associated with greater response rates with 50% of patients reporting an improvement after 26 week course. Overall, few of these studies were of high quality, as reported in recent systematic reviews with meta-analysis, with 1b level of evidence and grade of recommendations C [4–6]. According to AUA guidelines, PPS may be administered as second line oral medication [3].

Chondroitin sulfate and Hyaluronic acid. Many uncontrolled single-center studies including a small number of patients have been performed with the use of these agents in the treatment of IC/BPS, suggesting that both intravesical chondroitin sulfate and hyaluronic acid can improve symptoms in IC/PBS patients [26–29]. Indeed, in IC/BPS the concentration of these substances in the urothelium is reduced and urothelial permeability toward potassium compounds is increased, causing bladder pain. The potential benefit of chondroitin sulfate was detected by Nickel and co-workers in a randomized controlled study [30]. Although the study was not powered to show a significant difference between active therapy and vehicle control, many patients reported a clinically significant benefit with intravesical chondroitin sulfate treatment as compared with placebo. Intravesical chondroitin sulphate has been observed to induce side effects as dysuria, nausea, gastrointestinal upset, macular rash and urethritis in 77% of patients [26–30]. Also chondroitin sulfate and hyaluronic acid have been used alone or in combination with other pharmacological agents (i.e. heparin, lidocaine) and with bladder hydrodistension [4–6]. A positive and durable impact of HA therapy on IC/PBS symptoms was observed by Riedl and co-workers, with 85% patients reporting symptom improvement (> or =2 VAS units) [31]. HA with bladder hydrodistension, together with the addition of KCl and NaCl induced a 62.5% and 71.48% improvements on pain in the study of Daha and co-workers [32]. In the study of Shao et al. [33], HA alone or in combination with hydrodistention, lidocaine and heparin did not induce any improvement in pain, bladder capacity or urinary frequency.

Overall, the use of these GAG-like agents require additional clinical randomised controlled studies in order to better define which is their effect in the treatment of IC/BPS patients.

19.2.2 Antihistamines

The role of antihistamines in controlling symptoms of IC/BPS is still controversial. The histamine receptor antagonist *hydroxyzine* blocks the H1-receptor subtypes and inhibits the activation of mast cells. Previous studies reported an improvement in >90% of IC/BPS patients treated with this medication [4–6]. However, a more recent prospective, randomised controlled trial did not demonstrate any statistically significant improvement with hydroxyzine compared to a placebo [22].

The H2- receptor antagonist *cimetidine* has been observed to be effective in controlling IC/BPS symptoms in 71% of treated patients, with a dosage of 200 mg three times daily. A subsequent, 3- month follow up randomised controlled trial confirmed these previous results [34].

19.2.3 Antidepressants

To date there is enough evidence that *amitriptyline* increasing doses (from 25 to 100 mg) administered for some months is able to control pain and urgency in IC/BPS patients, as demonstrated by the study of van Opoven et al. [35]. In another high quality study, amitriptyline with different dosages and times of administration (increasing doses once daily from 10 to 75 mg for 12 weeks) with the addition of behavioural modification, showed a great effect size in ICSI and urinary frequency [36]. Importantly, amitriptyline is associated with high rates of significant side-effects, as dry mouth, dizziness and gastrointestinal problems, which limit the long term use of the substance. Nevertheless, both AUA and EAU recommended amitriptyline as a treatment option for IC/PBS patients [2, 3]. Other anti-depressant drugs potentially useful for the treatment of IC/BPS patients could be *doxepin, desipramine* and *duloxetine* [37], but the available data on their efficacy are still very limited.

19.2.4 Immunosuppressants and Corticosteroids

Cyclosporine A (CYA). CyA is a potent immunosuppressive agent used to decrease the risk of rejection after organ transplantation and to treat autoimmune conditions such as psoriasis, atopic dermatitis and rheumatoid arthritis [38]. It has been hypothesized that CyA binds to cyclophilins in T cells to antagonize the calcineurin mediated dephosphorylation of inactive nuclear factor of activated T cells, which is required for T cell activation [38]. One study compared CyA 1.5 mg/kg twice daily versus low dose PPS for 6 months in patients affected by IC/BPS [24]. A significantly higher response rate was detected with CyA (75% vs. 19%, $P < 0.05$), particularly on three outcomes (pain, frequency and IC Symptom Index). Mild adverse events were common in the CyA arm, and were reported by a total of 30 patients (among 32) compared to 18 (among 32) patients in the PPS arm. Significant adverse events (increased blood pressure and serum creatinine) were reported in the CyA arm. At 6 months patients were asked if they wanted to proceed with the current treatment. A total of 19 patients chose to continue on CyA treatment and 4 patients continued on PPS treatment.

Other potential immunosuppressive agents for IC/PBS could be *methotrexate and suplatast tosilate* [39, 40] but data on their therapeutic potential are to date really limited. With regards to the use of corticosteroids in patients with IC/BPS, AUA guidelines recommend that oral long-term glucocorticoid therapy should not be offered as treatment in patients with IC/BPS [3].

19.3 Emerging Targets

19.3.1 Anti-Nerve Growth Factor Treatment

It has been shown that nerve growth factor (NGF) is involved in inflammation, and allergic reaction, and altered neurological conditions in IC/BPS [41]. An immunohistological study reports that expression of NGF is increased in the bladder of IC/BPS patients [42]. Neurotrophic factors including NGF are also found in urine obtained from IC/BPS patients [43] and a recent meta-analysis study reported that urinary NGF could be a useful biomarker for the differential diagnosis of IC/BPS and overactive bladder as well as a predictive biomarker to help guide treatments [44]. Evans et al. [45] reported the clinical outcome of tanezumab, a monoclonal NGF neutralizing antibody for IC/BPS in phase II study. Tanezumab was administered intravenously in 68 patients with IC/BPS, and effective for self-reported pain and urinary urgency for 6 weeks compared to the placebo group, while voiding frequency and voided volume are not affected. However, serious adverse events were reported by another clinical trial of tanezumab for osteoarthritis, in which bone necrosis developed and total joint replacements were needed, and several clinical trials have since been terminated (www.clinicaltrials.gov). However, another human monoclonal antibody directed against NGF, fulranumab, did not show efficacy, but the authors did not exclude the possibility that the drug would provide clinical benefit in a larger study and/or specific populations [46]. Thus, these results provide the proof-of-concept evidence showing that NGF is an important pathophysiological factor inducing pain-related symptom in IC/BPS and that intervention of the NGF mechanism is effective for the treatment of IC/BPS; however, another local approach such as liposome-based intravesical therapy targeting NGF [47] should be developed to avoid systemic adverse events in future.

19.3.2 Intravesical Lidocaine Treatment

Local anesthetics such as lidocaine, which suppress neuronal excitation, have demonstrated properties that block the neuroinflammatory cycle associated with IC/BPS [48]. Intravesical lidocaine has been shown to be an effective treatment for IC/BPS. A clinical trial reported that alkalinized lidocaine and sodium bicarbonate relieve IC/BPS symptoms, as reported in the significant decrease of the GRA score, compared to the placebo (30% and 9.6%, respectively) [49]. The success rate is relatively higher than other intravesical drugs, but the post-therapeutic observation period is short; therefore, the treatment is also defined as an option in the AUA guideline [3].

The lidocaine-releasing intravesical system (LiRIS®) is a solid mini pellet, which encases lidocaine in a water-permeable flexible tube and releases lidocaine continuously [50]. In this open-label clinical trial without a placebo arm in 16 IC/BPS women with bladder pathologies such as Hunner lesions or glomerulations identified cystoscopically, clinically meaningful reductions in pain, urgency, voiding frequency, and disease questionnaires were seen after 14 days of LiRIS treatment. Cystoscopic examinations showed improvement on day 14 (day of removal) compared with day 1, including resolution of Hunner lesions in five of six subjects with baseline lesions. Extended follow-up suggests that the reduction in pain was maintained for several months after the device was removed [50].

These results of intravesical lidocaine treatment in IC/BPS patients suggest that; (1) lidocaine can reduce not only symptoms, but also neurogenic inflammation in the bladder by blocking nerve activity, (2) the bladder is a triggering organ of pain symptoms in the significant number of IC/BPS patients, especially when the bladder pathology is identified and (3) intravesical lidocaine administration would be useful as a diagnostic test to identify the patient population that is suitable for bladder-targeting therapies.

19.3.3 P2X3 Receptor Antagonist

Bladder distention releases ATP from the urothelium, and ATP activates P2X3 receptors in bladder afferents to modulate bladder activity evidenced by experimental studies of P2X3 knockout mice [51]. There is also evidence showing that the stimulatory ATP mechanism is upregulated in the bladder from IC/BPS patients because ATP release from urothelial cells in addition to urothelial expression of P2X3 ATP receptors are increased in IC/BPS patients [52–55]. A recent placebo-controlled clinical trial in 36 women treated with AF-219 and 38 women treated with placebo showed that patients treated with AF-219 for 4 weeks [56] had improvement in the key symptoms of IC/BPS such as pain scores, urinary urgency and in Global Response Assessment (GRA), compared to placebo-treated patients. There were 5 patients (4 in the AF-219 arm and 1 in the placebo arm) with Hunner lesions on cystoscopy. Thus, targeting the ATP and P2X receptor mechanism in the bladder would be a promising strategy for the treatment of IC/BPS with or without Hunner lesions.

19.3.4 AQX-1125, A Modulator of Immune/Inflammatory Processes

A new pharmaceutical class of compounds, represented by AQX-1125, has been recently introduced. AQX-1125 activates SH2-containing inositol-5′-phosphatase (SHIP1), modulating the PI3K pathway [57], which is involved in processes like cell growth, activation and immune/inflammatory conditions. Activation of SHIP1 has an anti-inflammatory effect by negatively regulating the PI3K pathway to reduce the immunological reaction [57]. AQX-1125 has been studied in a short-term, phase II, randomized, placebo controlled study, which included patients with moderate to severe IC/BPS, some with Hunner lesions (Aquinox Trial) [58]. Thirty-seven IC/BPS women were treated with the compound and 32 with placebo. Women treated with AQX-1125 showed a significant reduction in bladder pain and improvement of symptoms at 6 weeks compared to placebo-treated women [58].

It has been demonstrated that Hunner lesions show over-expression of genes related to immune and inflammatory responses, including helper T cell-related chemokines, whereas similar expression changes are not found in IC/BPS without Hunner lesion [59]. Thus, the anti-inflammatory treatment targeting the PI3K pathway could potentially be a useful strategy for the treatment of IC/BPS patients, especially when bladder inflammatory changes such as Hunner lesions are identified in the bladder.

19.3.4.1 Where Were We Off Base?

In the 1988 chapter, "the most urgent pharmacotherapeutic goal should be to make the patients symptom-free". Even if the ambitious goal is still valid, the current focus is on management of pain and its consequences. Various etiologies of IC/BPS have been postulated, which include urothelial dysfunction with increased permeability, alterations in growth factor expression, neurogenic inflammation with mast cell activation and increased NO levels, autoimmune reaction, infection, increased afferent activity and changes in CNS responses. In animal studies, blocking various proposed causes seems to be effective for the treatments of IC/BPS; however, the results in animal studies have not come to fruition in clinical trials. One of the reasons for the discrepancy could be the subtype of IC/BPS. The European Society for the Study of Interstitial Cystitis (ESSIC) proposed that Hunner's lesion, which is often called "ulcer", is not a typical chronic ulcer, but rather a distinctive inflammatory lesion presenting a characteristic deep rupture through the mucosa. Thus, IC/BPS with Hunner lesion might be a different entity from that without Hunner lesion [10], as similarly discussed 30 years ago by the same author [60]. An important question is whether the pain in the two conditions has different characteristics that would have therapeutic consequences. This does not seem to be the case. In a mail survey study of IC/BPS pain, including 749 women, Killinger et al. [61] focused on whether pain characteristics in women grouped by IC/BPS subtype would differ: They could not find any significant differences in pain characteristics between subtypes.

19.3.4.2 What Seminal Publications Changed Our Thinking?

As discussed by previous and recent publications by Fall et al. [10, 62], for the individualized therapy of IC/BPS, the Hunner type IC should separately be treated as a different phenotype from non-Hunner IC/BPS. The pathophysiology-based treatments of IC/BPS could be developed as shown by recent proof-of-cencept clinical trials of anti-NGF treatment [45, 46], ATP receptor antagonist [56] and SHIP1 inhibitor [58].

19.3.4.3 Where Do We Go from Here?

The heterogeneity of patient populations in IC/BPS may be one of the reasons why many drugs fail to demonstrate overall efficacy. Thus, the key for the future success in development of effective pharmacotherapies of IC/BPS would be the appropriate selection of target population(s) among IC/BPS patients based on phenotyping of the disease. When the bladder-centric therapies are selected, the cystoscopic evaluation of the existence of Hunner lesion in participants of clinical trials increases the chance of successful outcomes. We consider that it is important to draw a distinction between these two conditions because the prevalence of Hunner lesion among IC/BPS patients is higher than previously expected, and reaches up to 50% of IC/BPS patients [10, 62, 63]. In addition, glomerulations, which are defined as multiple petechia-like hemorrhages on bladder distension, have been used as a diagnostic criterion for IC/BPS; however, the specificity of glomerulations is in question as they are seen not only in IC/BPS but also in other conditions [64]. Therefore, the additional approaches such as cystoscopic evaluation with a narrow band imaging system would be necessary to increase the rate and accuracy of detection of bladder pathological changes in IC/BPS [65]. In addition, Nickel et al. [9] proposed the individualized therapeutic strategies based on the phenotype of IC/BPS symptoms, which is classified by the UPOINT categorization (urinary, psychosocial, organ-specific, infection, neurologic or non-bladder, and tenderness of pelvic floor. Taken together, we presume that standardized classification of IC/BPS is important for the evaluation of efficacy of new drug treatments.

References

1. Rovner E, Propert KJ, Brensinger C, Wein AJ, Foy M, Kirkemo A, Landis JR, Kusek JW, Nyberg LM. Treatments used in women with interstitial cystitis: the interstitial cystitis data base (ICDB) study experience. The Interstitial Cystitis Data Base Study Group. Urology. 2000;56(6):940–5.
2. Engeler DS, Baranowski AP, Dinis-Oliveira P, Elneil S, Hughes J, Messelink EJ, van Ophoven A, Williams AC, European Association of Urology. The 2013 EAU guidelines on chronic pelvic pain: is management of chronic pelvic pain a habit, a philosophy, or a science? 10 years of development. Eur Urol. 2013;64:431–9.
3. Hanno PM, Burks DA, Clemens JQ, Dmochowski RR, Erickson D, Fitzgerald MP, Forrest JB, Gordon B, Gray M, Mayer RD, Newman D, Nyberg L Jr, Payne CK, Wesselmann U, Faraday MM, Interstitial Cystitis Guidelines Panel of the American Urological Association Education and Research, Inc. AUA guideline for the diagnosis and treatment of interstitial cystitis/bladder pain syndrome. J Urol. 2011;185:2162–70.
4. Giannantoni A, Bini V, Dmochowski R, Hanno P, Nickel JC, Proietti S, Wyndaele JJ. Contemporary management of the painful bladder: a systematic review. Eur Urol. 2012;61:29–53.
5. Davis NF, Brady CM, Creagh T. Interstitial cystitis/painful bladder syndrome: epidemiology, pathophysiology and evidence-based treatment options. Eur J Obstet Gynecol Reprod Biol. 2014;175:30–7.
6. Pazin C, Moreira de Souza Mitidieri A, Moreira Silva AP, Ferreira Gurian MB, Poli-Neto OB, Rosa-e-Silva JC. Treatment of bladder pain syndrome and interstitial cystitis: a systematic review. Int Urogynecol J. 2016;27:697–708.
7. van de Merwe JP, Nordling J, Bouchelouche P, et al. Diagnostic criteria, classification, and nomenclature for painful bladder syndrome/interstitial cystitis: an ESSIC proposal. Eur Urol. 2008;53(1):60–7.
8. Ogawa T, Ishizuka O, Ueda T, Tyagi P, Chancellor MB, Yoshimura N. Current and emerging drugs for

interstitial cystitis/bladder pain syndrome (IC/BPS). Expert Opin Emerg Drugs. 2015;20(4):555–70.
9. Fall M, Logadottir Y, Peeker R. Interstitial cystitis is bladder pain syndrome with Hunner's lesion. Int J Urol. 2014;21(Suppl 1):79–82.
10. Nickel JC, Irvine-Bird K, Jianbo L, et al. Phenotype-directed management of interstitial cystitis/bladder pain syndrome. Urology. 2014 Jul;84(1):175–9.
11. Hurst RE. Structure, function and pathology of proteoglycans and glycosaminoglycans in the urinary tract. World J Urol. 1994;12:3–10.
12. Emtage J, Morales A, Heaton JPW, Perez-Marrero R. Heparin in the treatment of interstitial cystitis. J Urol. 1985;133:168.
13. Morales A, Emerson L, Nickel JC, Lundie M. Intravesical hyaluronic acid in the treatment of refractory interstitial cystitis. J Urol. 1996;156:45–9.
14. Bade JJ, Laseur M, Nieuwenburg LT, van der Weele LT, Mensink HJ. A placebo-controlled study of intravesical Pentosanpolysulfate for the treatment of interstitial cystitis. Br J Urol. 1997;79:168–71.
15. Parsons CL, Schmidt JD, Pollen JJ. Successful treatment of interstitial cystitis with sodium pentosan polysulfate. J Urol. 1983;130:51–3.
16. Hanno PM. Analysis of long-term Elmiron therapy for interstitial cystitis. Urology. 1997;49(5A Suppl):93–9.
17. Jepsen JV, Sall M, Rhodes PR, Schmidt D, Messing E, Bruskewitz RC. Long term experience with pentosanpolysulfate in interstitial cystitis. Urology. 1998;51:381–7.
18. Nickel JC, Kaufman DM, Zhang HF, Wan GJ, Sand PK. Time to initiation of pentosan polysulfate sodium treatment after interstitial cystitis diagnosis: effect on symptom improvement. Urology. 2008;71:57–61.
19. Sand PK, Kaufman DM, Evans RJ, Zhang HF, Alan Fisher DL, Nickel JC. Association between response to pentosan polysulfate sodium therapy for interstitial cystitis and patient questionnaire-based treatment satisfaction. Curr Med Res Opin. 2008;24:2259–64.
20. Chuang YC, Lee WC, Lee WC, Chiang PH. Intravesical liposome versus oral pentosan polysulfate for interstitial cystitis/painful bladder syndrome. J Urol. 2009;182:1393–400.
21. Parsons CL, Benson G, Childs SJ, Hanno P, Sant GR, Webster G. A quantitatively controlled method to study prospectively interstitial cystitis and demonstrate the efficacy of pentosanpolysulfate. J Urol. 1993;150:845–8.
22. Sant GR, Propert KJ, Hanno PM, et al. A pilot clinical trial of oral pentosan polysulfate and oral hydroxyzine in patients with interstitial cystitis. J Urol. 2003;170:810–5.
23. Nickel JC, Barkin J, Forrest J, et al. Randomized, double-blind, dose ranging study of pentosan polysulfate sodium for interstitial cystitis. Urology. 2005;65:654–8.
24. Sairanen J, Tammela TLJ, Leppilahti M, et al. Cyclosporine A and pentosanpolysulfate sodium for the treatment of interstitial cystitis: a randomized comparative study. J Urol. 2005;174:2235–8.
25. Davis EL, El Khoudary SR, Talbott EO, Davis J, Regan LJ. Safety and efficacy of the use of intravesical and oral pentosan polysulfate sodium for interstitial cystitis: a randomized double-blind clinical trial. J Urol. 2008;179:177–85.
26. Sorensen RB. Chondroitin sulphate in the treatment of interstitial cystitis and chronic inflammatory disease of the urinary bladder. Eur Urol Suppl. 2003;2(4):16–8.
27. Steinhoff G. The efficacy of chondroitin sulphate in treating interstitial cystitis. Eur Urol Suppl. 2003;14-16(10):2.
28. Nickel JC, Egerdie B, Downey J, Singh R, Skehan A, Carr L, Irvine-Bird K. A real-life multi-centre clinical practice study to evaluate the efficacy and safety of intravesical chondroitin sulfate for the treatment of interstitial cystitis. BJU Int 2008;103:56–6.
29. Nordling J, van Ophoven A. Intravesical Glysosaminoglycan replenishment with chondroitin sulfate in chronic forms of cystitis. Arzneimittelforschung. 2008;58:328–35.
30. Nickel JC, Egerdie RB, Steinhoff G, Palmer B, Hanno P. A multicenter, randomized, double-blind, parallel group pilot evaluation of the efficacy and safety of intravesical sodium chondroitin sulfate versus vehicle control in patients with interstitial cystitis/painful bladder syndrome. Urology. 2010;76:804–9.
31. Riedl CR, Engelhardt PF, Daha KL, Morakis N, Pflüger H. Hyaluronan treatment of interstitial cystitis/painful bladder syndrome. Int Urogynecol J Pelvic Floor Dysfunct. 2008;19:717–21.
32. Daha LK, Riedl CR, Lazar D, Hohlbrugger G, Pflüger H. Do cystometric findings predict the results of intravesical hyaluronic acid in women with interstitial cystitis? Eur Urol. 2005;47:393–7.
33. Shao Y, Shen ZJ, RuiWB ZWL. Intravesical instillation of hyaluronic acid prolonged the effect of bladder hydrodistention in patients with severe interstitial cystitis. J Urol. 2010;75:547–50.
34. Thilagarajah R, Witherow RO, Walker MM. Oral cimetidine gives effective symptom relief in painful bladder disease: a prospective, randomized, double-blind placebo-controlled trial. BJU Int. 2001;87:207–12.
35. van Ophoven A, Pokupic S, Heinecke A, Hertle L. A prospective, randomized, placebo controlled, double-blind study ofamitriptyline for the treatment of interstitial cystitis. J Urol. 2004;172:533–6.
36. Foster HE, Hanno PM, Nickel JC, et al. Effect of amitriptyline on symptoms in treatment naive patients with interstitial cystitis/ painful bladder syndrome. J Urol. 2010;183:1853–8.
37. van Ophoven A, Hertle L. The dual serotonin and noradrenaline reuptake inhibitor duloxetine for the treatment of interstitial cystitis: results of an observational study. J Urol. 2007;177:552–5.
38. Kapturczak MH, Meier-Kriesche HU, Kaplan B. Pharmacology of calcineurin antagonists. Transplant Proc. 2004;36(2 Suppl):25S–32S.
39. Moran PA, Dwyer PL, Carey MP, Maher CF, Radford NJ. Oral methotrexate in the management of refrac-

tory interstitial cystitis. Aust N Z J Obstet Gynaecol. 1999;39(4):468–71.
40. Ueda T, Tamaki M, Ogawa O, Yamauchi T, Yoshimura N. Improvement of interstitial cystitis symptoms and problems that developed during treatment with oral IPD-1151T. J Urol. 2000;164:1917–20.
41. Ochodnicky P, Cruz CD, Yoshimura N, Cruz F. Neurotrophins as regulators of urinary bladder function. Nat Rev Urol. 2012;9(11):628–37.
42. Lowe EM, Anand P, Terenghi G, et al. Increased nerve growth factor levels in the urinary bladder of women with idiopathic sensory urgency and interstitial cystitis. Br J Urol. 1997;79(4):572–7.
43. Okragly AJ, Niles AL, Saban R, et al. Elevated tryptase, nerve growth factor, neurotrophin-3 and glial cell line-derived neurotrophic factor levels in the urine of interstitial cystitis and bladder cancer patients. J Urol. 1999;161(2):438–41. discussion 41-2
44. HC Q, Zhang W, Yan S, et al. Urinary nerve growth factor could be a biomarker for interstitial cystitis/painful bladder syndrome: a meta-analysis. PLoS One. 2014;9(9):e106321.
45. Evans RJ, Moldwin RM, Cossons N, et al. Proof of concept trial of tanezumab for the treatment of symptoms associated with interstitial cystitis. J Urol. 2011;185(5):1716–21.
46. Wang H, Russell LJ, Kelly KM, Wang S, Thipphawong J. Fulranumab in patients with interstitial cystitis/bladder pain syndrome: observations from a randomized, double-blind, placebo-controlled study. BMC Urol. 2017;17(1):2.
47. Tyagi P, Kashyap M, Majima T, Kawamorita N, Yoshizawa T, Yoshimura N. Intravesical liposome therapy for interstitial cystitis. Int J Urol. 2017;24(4):267–71.
48. Henry RA, Morales A, Cahill CM. Beyond a simple anesthetic effect: lidocaine in the diagnosis and treatment of interstitial cystitis/bladder pain syndrome. Urology. 2015;85(5):1025–33.
49. Nickel JC, Moldwin R, Lee S, et al. Intravesical alkalinized lidocaine (PSD597) offers sustained relief from symptoms of interstitial cystitis and painful bladder syndrome. BJU Int. 2009;103(7):910–8.
50. Nickel JC, Jain P, Shore N, et al. Continuous intravesical lidocaine treatment for interstitial cystitis/bladder pain syndrome: safety and efficacy of a new drug delivery device. Sci Transl Med. 2012;4(143):143ra00.
51. Cockayne DA, Hamilton SG, Zhu QM, et al. Urinary bladder hyporeflexia and reduced pain-related behaviour in P2X3-deficient mice. Nature. 2000;407(6807):1011–5.
52. Sun Y, Chai TC. Effects of dimethyl sulphoxide and heparin on stretch-activated ATP release by bladder urothelial cells from patients with interstitial cystitis. BJU Int. 2002;90(4):381–5.
53. Sun Y, Keay S, De Deyne PG, et al. Augmented stretch activated adenosine triphosphate release from bladder uroepithelial cells in patients with interstitial cystitis. J Urol. 2001;166(5):1951–6.
54. Sun Y, Chai TC. Up-regulation of P2X3 receptor during stretch of bladder urothelial cells from patients with interstitial cystitis. J Urol. 2004;171(1):448–52.
55. Sun Y, Chai TC. Augmented extracellular ATP signaling in bladder urothelial cells from patients with interstitial cystitis. Am J Physiol Cell Physiol. 2006;290(1):C27–34.
56. Moldwin R, Kitt M, Mangel J, Beyer R, Hanno P, Butera P, Ford A. A phase 2 study in women with interstitial cystitis/bladder pain syndrome (IC/BPS) of the novel P2X3 antagonist AF-219 (Abstract #23), 45th International Continence Society (ICS) Annual Meeting, Montreal, Canada, 2015.
57. Stenton GR, Mackenzie LF, Tam P, et al. Characterization of AQX-1125, a small-molecule SHIP1 activator: Part 1. Effects on inflammatory cell activation and chemotaxis in vitro and pharmacokinetic characterization in vivo. Br J Pharmacol. 2013;168(6):1506–18.
58. Nickel JC, Egerdie B, Davis E, Evans R, Mackenzie L, Shrewsbury SB. A phase II study of the efficacy and safety of the novel oral SHIP1 activator AQX-1125 in subjects with moderate to severe interstitial cystitis/bladder pain syndrome. J Urol. 2016;196(3):747–54.
59. Ogawa T, Homma T, Igawa Y, et al. CXCR3 binding chemokine and TNFSF14 over expression in bladder urothelium of patients with ulcerative interstitial cystitis. J Urol. 2010;183(3):1206–12.
60. Fall M, Johansson SL, Aldenborg F. Chronic interstitial cystitis: a heterogeneous syndrome. J Urol. 1987;137(1):35–8.
61. Killinger KA, Boura JA, Peters KM. Pain in interstitial cystitis/bladder pain syndrome: do characteristics differ in ulcerative and non-ulcerative subtypes? Int Urogynecol J. 2013;24(8):1295–301.
62. Fall M, Baranowski AP, Elneil S, et al. EAU guidelines on chronic pelvic pain. Eur Urol. 2010;57(1):35–48.
63. Logadottir Y, Fall M, Kabjorn-Gustafsson C, et al. Clinical characteristics differ considerably between phenotypes of bladder pain syndrome/interstitial cystitis. Scand J Urol Nephrol. 2012;46(5):365–70.
64. Wennevik GE, Meijlink JM, Hanno P, Nordling J. The role of glomerulations in bladder pain syndrome: a review. J Urol. 2016;195(1):19–25.
65. Ueda T, Nakagawa M, Okamura M, et al. New cystoscopic diagnosis for interstitial cystitis/painful bladder syndrome using narrow-band imaging system. Int J Urol. 2008;15(12):1039–43.

Intravesical Therapy of Interstitial Cystitis

20

Philip Hanno

20.1 What Did We Get Right?

Flashback to 1989. Bladder Pain Syndrome/ Interstitial Cystitis was treated with a variety of off-label therapies, but the standard treatment against which all therapies were measured was intravesical lavage. Dimethyl sulfoxide (DMSO) had been approved a decade earlier (1978) for treatment of interstitial cystitis and remains to this day the only approved intravesical medication for the disorder by the Food and Drug Administration (FDA). Its use for this condition can be credited to Bruce Stewart of the Cleveland Clinic who persisted with an intravesical trial after failing in a transdermal clinical study of refractory patients in the mid-1960's. It would be 1996 before sodium pentosan polysulfate became only the second approved medication and sole oral approved therapy for the syndrome.

DMSO, a colorless and odorless organic solvent, would have difficulty attracting a pharmaceutical company to invest in therapeutic trials were it to have come to market today. The garlic odor which is the hallmark of use (possibly resulting from a nonolfactory activation of TRPAA1 receptors [1] makes doing a blinded, placebo controlled trial almost an impossibility, and approval from regulatory authorities unlikely.

P. Hanno
Stanford University School of Medicine, Stanford, CA, USA
e-mail: philip.hanno@stanford.edu

The chapter Dr. Wein and I co-authored in 1989 also discusses two intravesical therapies that are rarely if ever used three decades later.

Silver nitrate was first used in the mid nineteenth century for the symptoms of bladder pain syndrome. It was championed at the Mayo Clinic and the evidence of efficacy is noted in the original chapter. It has been used, often unsuccessfully, for the treatment of hemorrhagic cystitis [2]. Pain on instillation which may require sedation, the risk of bladder fibrosis retroperitoneal and renal damage if bladder perforation or reflux are present at the time of administration [3], and the risk of argyrosis [4] have limited if not completely removed it from the BPS armamentarium.

Clorpactin WCS 90 was successfully used in 1855 for the symptoms of BPS. It gained adherents after a number of positive publications in the twentieth century culminating in its dominant position in a classic and seminal publication on interstitial cystitis by Ed Messing and Tom Stamey out of Stanford in 1978. It was in this journal article that glomerulations were established as a keystone in diagnosis in patients with symptoms of bladder pain and voiding dysfunction. A follow up paper from the Stanford group indicating the possibility of ureteral fibrosis in patients with reflux served as a cautionary warning that a cystogram should be performed prior to instillation to rule out this possibility. The last publication I could find on clorpactin, and the only one after 1970, was by Kreder et al. in 2001 indicating that the mechanism of action might be through release of calcitonin

P.M. Hanno et al. (eds.), *Bladder Pain Syndrome – An Evolution*,
https://doi.org/10.1007/978-3-319-61449-6_20

gene-related peptide [5]. It's not clear why this relatively effective intravesical therapy has so fallen out of favor. I think that patients are not predisposed to essentially putting a bleach solution into their bladders. Sodium oxychlorosene, the generic form of the brand, is essentially a relative of Dakin's solution, an antiseptic solution developed during World War I to treat infected wounds by combining water, baking soda and bleach. Urologists tend to shy away from unapproved therapies that require anesthesia to administer and can cause damage if extravasation or reflux is present. Information on Clorpactin WCS-90 is available from the manufacturer at www.u-g.com/info.download.php?id=33.

20.2 What Did We Get Wrong?

While therapeutically targeting the bladder was certainly reasonable, and remains so today, we did not realize that the disease in many patients has a more decentralized focus and in many patients is a part of a broader chronic pain syndrome that may not respond to treatments focused primarily on the bladder. We did not do randomized placebo-controlled trials to prove efficacy, largely because such trials could not easily be blinded, and thus today are still trying to estimate efficacy of many of these older intravesical solutions without the data necessary to make a valid judgement. Though intravesical and subcutaneous heparin had been considered (see below), intravesical instillation of glycosaminoglycans as a standard treatment option was years away. We had not considered direct intradetrusor application of therapies three decades ago.

20.3 What Seminal Publications Changed Our Thinking?

Perez-Marrero R, Emerson LE, Maharajh DO, et al.. Prolongation of response to DMSO by heparin maintenance. Urology. 1993;41 (suppl):64–6.

Mayer R, Propert KJ, Peters KM, Payne CK, Zhang Y, Burks D, et al. A randomized controlled trial of intravesical bacillus calmette-guerin for treatment refractory interstitial cystitis. J Urol. 2005;173(4):1186–91.

Payne CK, Mosbaugh PG, Forrest JB, Evans RJ, Whitmore KE, Antoci JP, et al. Intravesical resiniferatoxin for the treatment of interstitial cystitis: a randomized, double-blind, placebo controlled trial. J Urol. 2005;173(5):1590–4.

Nickel JC, Moldwin R, Lee S, Davis EL, Henry RA, Wyllie MG. Intravesical alkalinized lidocaine (PSD597) offers sustained relief from symptoms of interstitial cystitis and painful bladder syndrome. BJU Int. 2009;103(7): 910–8.

Madersbacher H, van Ophoven A, van Kerrebroeck PE. GAG layer replenishment therapy for chronic forms of cystitis with intravesical glycosaminoglycans—a review. Neurourol Urodyn. 2013;32(1):9–18.

Throughout the world, interest in developing new intravesical therapies for BPS has mushroomed over the last few decades since the publication of Interstitial Cystitis. The potential for a high ratio of efficacy to side effects has interested pharmaceutical companies and clinical researchers. One would expect these direct bladder therapies to be most effective in patients with primarily bladder pain rather than in those with a generalized pain disorder manifest by the presence of multiple pain syndromes. Exogenous glycosaminoglycans have been the prominent treatment modality, though none have garnered an FDA indication for BPS.

Exogenous glycosaminoglycans have been shown to be effective in providing an epithelial permeability barrier in bladders in which the epithelium has been injured with protamine [6]. ***Heparin***, which can mimic the activity of the bladder's own mucopolysaccharide lining [7], has anti-inflammatory effects as well as actions which inhibit fibroblast proliferation, angiogenesis, and smooth muscle cell proliferation. Because of its numerous effects, the possibility that heparin could be used for therapeutic reasons other than the control of coagulation has been the subject of much inquiry and speculation [8]. Weaver first reported intravesical heparin for IC treatment [9]. Given intravesically, there is virtually no systemic absorption, even in an inflamed bladder [10]. While uncontrolled studies suggested some beneficial effect for subcutaneous administration [11, 12], the obvious risks of anticoagulation and osteoporosis have prevented this form of administration from undergoing further trials and general usage. Ten thousand units can be administered intravesically in sterile water either alone or with DMSO at varying intervals with good results reported [13, 14]. Kuo reported 50% or more improvement in the International Prostate Symptom Score in 29 of 40 women with IC treated with 25,000 units intravesically twice weekly for 3 months [15].

Parsons has used daily intravesical doses of 40,000 units of heparin in 20 cc sterile water administered by the patient daily and held for 30–60 min. "Reasonable improvement of symptoms" can be expected between 6 months and 2 years after starting therapy [16]. Adding alkalinized lidocaine to the heparin instillation provides better pain relief [17]. The addition of 8 mL of 2% lidocaine and 4 mL of 8.4% sodium bicarbonate may improve results [18]. In fact, a combination of 200 mg lidocaine with 8.4% sodium bicarbonate (10 mL total solution) *without* heparin showed a 30% response rate 3 days after completion of daily intravesical administration for 5 days and was statistically superior to a placebo cocktail [19]. A Japanese study reported high success rates with weekly intravesical instillation of 20,000 units heparin with 5 mL of 4% lidocaine and 25 mL of 7% sodium bicarbonate for 12 weeks [20]. Intravesical alkalinized lidocaine and heparin has been proposed as a treatment for symptom flare [21].

Other glycosaminoglycans administered intravesically include pentosanpolysulfate, hyaluronic acid, chondroitin sulfate, and combinations of hyaluronic acid and chondroitin sulfate [22–26]. While non-placebo controlled trials suggest efficacy, no definitive large scale randomized placebo controlled trials have been reported to show benefit, and none have been approved for a BPS indication in the United States. A comprehensive analysis of glycosaminoglycan layer replenishment therapy with intravesical glycosaminoglycans concluded that despite the fact that GAG intravesical therapy has been in use for over two decades, most of the studies are uncontrolled, poorly done, and with a small number of patients. Large-scale randomized controlled trials are urgently needed to underline the benefit of this type of therapy. Distinct patient groups (well phenotyped) need to be confirmed by definitive diagnostic findings [27]. Another review sadly concludes that "randomized controlled trials have suggested the GAG analogues are at best as good as placebo" [28].

The use of intravesical **bacillus Calmette-Guerin (BCG)** for interstitial cystitis was first reported by Zeidman and colleagues [29]. A subsequent randomized, prospective, double-blind, placebo controlled trial of 30 patients treated weekly for 6 weeks and followed for a mean of 8 months noted a 60% response rate compared to a 27% placebo response [30]. Surprisingly, BCG was tolerated as well as placebo. Even more surprisingly, eight of nine BCG responders continued to have an excellent response in all parameters measured at 27 months of follow-up [31]. It is unclear how BCG achieved this result, but immunologic and/or anti-inflammatory mechanisms have been postulated [32]. A double-blind crossover Swedish study comparing DMSO to BCG failed to substantiate BCG efficacy [33].

A large multicenter randomized controlled trial by NIDDK comparing BCG to placebo found a 12% response rate for placebo compared to a 21% response for BCG. Placebo responders in the trial had the same durability of response (up to 68 weeks) as the BCG responders [34]. In a follow-up open label phase of the trial, the response rate was 18% in both the group originally randomized to BCG and the group initially randomized to placebo, indicating a second course of therapy does not improve response rate [35]. The small response rate in the RCT failed to reach statistical significance at the $p = 0.05$ level, and this large study of 265 patients suggests that **BCG has no place in the treatment of moderate to severe BPS/IC** [36].

Resiniferatoxin (RTX), an ultra-potent analogue of capsaicin appears to have similar effects with less of the acute pain and irritation associated with capsaicin application. Both compounds have been tested intravesically for the relief of bladder instability and hyperreflexia [37]. Clinical trials for the use of these compounds in bladder pain, urgency/frequency could show this to be a new and viable treatment modality in the future, but **current data on efficacy in BPS are**

lacking [38–40]. A phase 2 safety and proof of concept multicenter, placebo-controlled trial conducted by ICOS Corporation of Bothell, WA found no significant efficacy of a single intravesical administration RTX compared with placebo, although no safety issues were identified [41]. RTX and hydrodistention was effective in relieving the pain of BPS when compared to hydrodistention alone, but was not effective in improving lower urinary tract symptoms [42]. Studies using other concentrations and multiple administrations may be worthwhile [43].

Liposomes, vesicals composed of concentric phospholipid bilayers separated by aqueous compartments, adsorb onto cell surfaces and fuse with cells. They can be used for drug delivery and gene therapy. They are currently in testing as an intravesical therapy for BPS [44, 45].

20.4 Where Do We Go from Here?

Intravesical therapy could be both diagnostic and therapeutic, helping us to decide in which patients the symptoms are mainly related to the bladder and in whom that is too narrow a therapeutic target. Patients with predominantly chronic central sensitization and those with primary pelvic floor dysfunction should not respond well to bladder-centric therapy. We desperately need to subject all therapies, and glycosaminoglycans in particular, to placebo-controlled trials to know whether they are truly effective. Better phenotyping will enable us to identify groups who are most likely to respond to such treatments. Development of drug delivery devices that can be placed in the bladder to slowly administer intravesical therapies and then dissolve and be voided out would be ideal for administering treatments for this disease and other primary bladder disorders.

References

1. Lübbert M, Kyereme J, Schöbel N, Beltrán L, Wetzel CH, Hatt H. Transient receptor potential channels encode volatile chemicals sensed by rat trigeminal ganglion neurons. PLoS One. 2013;8(10):e77998.
2. Montgomery BD, Boorjian SA, Ziegelmann MJ, Joyce DD, Linder BJ. Intravesical silver nitrate for refractory hemorrhagic cystitis. Turk J Urol. 2016;42(3):197–201.
3. Jerkins GR, Noe HN, Hill DE. An unusual complication of silver nitrate treatment of hemorrhagic cystitis: case report. J Urol. 1986;136(2):456–8.
4. Kojima Y, Uchida K, Takiuchi H, Wakatsuki A, Sakurai T, Fujita Y, et al. Argyrosis of the urinary tract after silver nitrate instillation: report of a case. Hinyokika Kiyo. 1993;39(1):41–4.
5. Kreder K, Lutgendorf S, Knopf MA, McGillis JP. Chlorpactin instillation releases calcitonin gene-related peptide in interstitial cystitis patients. Urology. 2001;57(6 Suppl 1):128–9.
6. Nickel JC, Downey J, Morales A, Emerson L, Clark J. Relative efficacy of various exogenous glycosaminoglycans in providing a bladder surface permeablility barrier. J Urol. 1998;160:612–4.
7. Hanno PM, Fritz R, Wein AJ. Heparin as an antibacterial agent in rabbit bladder. Urology. 1978;12:411–5.
8. Lane DA, Adams L. Non-anticoagulant uses of heparin. N Engl J Med. 1993;329:129–30.
9. Weaver RG, Dougherty TF, Natoli CA. Recent concepts of interstitial cystitis. J Urol. 1963;89:377–83.
10. Caulfield J, Phillips R, Steinhardt G. Intravesical heparin instillation: is there systemic absorption? J Urol. 1995;153:289A.
11. Lose G, Frandsen B, Hojensgard JC, Jespersen J, Astrup T. Chronic interstitial cystitis: increased levels of eosinophil cationic protein in serum and urine and an ameliorating effect of subcutaneous heparin. Scand J Urol Nephrol. 1983;17(2):159–61.
12. Lose G, Jespersen J, Frandsen B, Hojensgard JC, Astrup T. Subcutaneous heparin in the treatment of interstitial cystitis. Scand J Urol Nephrol. 1985;19(1):27–9.
13. Perez-Marrero R, Emerson LE, Maharajh DO, et al. Prolongation of response to DMSO by heparin maintenance. Urology. 1993;41(suppl):64–6.
14. Parsons CL, Housley T, Schmidt JD, Lebow D. Treatment of interstitial cystitis with intravesical heparin. Br J Urol. 1994;73(5):504–7.
15. Kuo HC. Urodynamic results of intravesical heparin therapy for women with frequency urgency syndrome and interstitial cystitis. J Formos Med Assoc. 2001;100(5):309–14.
16. Parsons CL. Interstitial cystitis: new concepts in pathogenesis, diagnosis, and management. AUA News. 5(4):20–31.
17. Parsons CL. Successful downregulation of bladder sensory nerves with combination of heparin and alkalinized lidocaine in patients with interstitial cystitis. Urology. 2005;65(1):45–8.
18. Welk BK, Teichman JM. Dyspareunia response in patients with interstitial cystitis treated with intravesical lidocaine, bicarbonate, and heparin. Urology. 2008;71(1):67–70.
19. Nickel JC, Moldwin R, Lee S, Davis EL, Henry RA, Wyllie MG. Intravesical alkalinized lidocaine (PSD597) offers sustained relief from symptoms of

interstitial cystitis and painful bladder syndrome. BJU Int. 2009;103(7):910–8.
20. Nomiya A, Naruse T, Niimi A, Nishimatsu H, Kume H, Igawa Y, Homma Y. On- and post-treatment symptom relief by repeated instillations of heparin and alkalized lidocaine in interstitial cystitis. Int J Urol. 2013;20(11):1118–22.
21. Parsons CL, Koziol JA, Proctor JG, Zupkas P, Argade S. Heparin and alkalinized lidocaine versus alkalinized lidocaine for treatment of interstitial cystitis symptoms. Can J Urol. 2015;22(2):7739–44.
22. Gülpınar O, Kayış A, Süer E, Gökçe Mİ, Güçlü AG, Arıkan N. Clinical comparision of intravesical hyaluronic acid and hyaluronic acid-chondroitin sulphate therapy for patients with bladder pain syndrome/interstitital cystitis. Can Urol Assoc J. 2014;8(9–10):E610–4.
23. Cervigni M. Interstitial cystitis/bladder pain syndrome and glycosaminoglycans replacement therapy. Transl Androl Urol. 2015;4(6):638–42.
24. Pyo JS, Cho WJ. Systematic review and meta-analysis of intravesical hyaluronic acid and hyaluronic acid/chondroitin sulfate instillation for interstitial cystitis/painful bladder syndrome. Cell Physiol Biochem. 2016;39(4):1618–25.
25. Lazzeri M, Hurle R, Casale P, Buffi N, Lughezzani G, Fiorini G, et al. Managing chronic bladder diseases with the administration of exogenous glycosaminoglycans: an update on the evidence. Ther Adv Urol. 2016;8(2):91–9.
26. Cervigni M, Sommariva M, Tenaglia R. A randomized open label, multicenter study of the efficacy and safety of intravesical hyaluronic acid and chondroitin sulfate versus dimethly sulfoxide in women with bladder pain syndrome/interstitial cystitis. Neurourol Urodyn. 2017;36(4):1178–86.
27. Madersbacher H, van Ophoven A, van Kerrebroeck PE. GAG layer replenishment therapy for chronic forms of cystitis with intravesical glycosaminoglycans--a review. Neurourol Urodyn. 2013;32(1):9–18.
28. Chintea CL, Belal M. Is there enough evidence for the use of intravesical instillations of glycosaminoglycan analogues in interstitial cystitis? BJU Int. 2013;111(2):192–3.
29. Zeidman EJ, Helfrick B, Pollard C, Thompson IM. Bacillus calmette-guerin immunotherapy for refractory interstitial cystitis. Urology. 1994;43(1):121–4.
30. Peters K, Diokno A, Steinert B, Yuhico M, Mitchell B, Krohta S, et al. The efficacy of intravesical tice strain bacillus calmette-guerin in the treatment of interstitial cystitis: a double-blind, prospective, placebo controlled trial. J Urol. 1997;157(6):2090–4.
31. Peters KM, Diokno AC, Steinert BW, Gonzalez JA. The efficacy of intravesical bacillus calmette-guerin in the treatment of interstitial cystitis: long-term followup. J Urol. 1998;159(5):1483–6.
32. Peters KM, Diokno AC, Steinert BW. Preliminary study on urinary cytokine levels in interstitial cystitis: does intravesical bacille calmette-guerin treat interstitial cystitis by altering the immune profile in the bladder? Urology. 1999;54(3):450–3.
33. Peeker R, Haghsheno MA, Holmang S, Fall M. Intravesical bacillus calmette-guerin and dimethyl sulfoxide for treatment of classic and nonulcer interstitial cystitis: a prospective, randomized double-blind study. J Urol. 2000;164(6):1912–5.
34. Propert K, Mayer R, Nickel C, Peters K, Teal V, Burks D, et al. Followup of patients with interstitial cystitis responsive to treatment with intravesical bacillus calmette-guerin or placebo. J Urol. 2008;179(2):552–5.
35. Propert KJ, Mayer R, Nickel JC, Payne CK, Peters KM, Teal V, et al. Did patients with interstitial cystitis who failed to respond to initial treatment with bacillus calmette-guerin or placebo in a randomized clinical trial benefit from a second course of open label bacillus calmette-guerin? J Urol. 2007;178(3 Pt 1):886–90.
36. Mayer R, Propert KJ, Peters KM, Payne CK, Zhang Y, Burks D, et al. A randomized controlled trial of intravesical bacillus calmette-guerin for treatment refractory interstitial cystitis. J Urol. 2005;173(4):1186–91.
37. Chancellor MB, de Groat WC. Intravesical capsaicin and resiniferatoxin therapy: spicing up the ways to treat the overactive bladder. J Urol. 1999;162:3–11.
38. Lazzeri M, Beneforti P, Benaim G, Maggi CA, Lecci A, Turini D. Intravesical capsaicin for treatment of severe bladder pain: a randomized placebo controlled study. J Urol. 1996;156:947–52.
39. Lazzeri M, Beneforti P, Turini D, Barbagli G, Palminteri E. Single dose of intravesical resiniferatoxin for the treatment of interstitial cystitis -- preliminary results of a randomised controlled study. J Urol. 2000;163S:60.
40. Cruz F, Guimaraes M, Silva C, Rio ME, Coimbra A, Reis M. Desensitization of bladder sensory fibers by intravesical capsaicin has long lasting clinical and urodynamic effects in patients with hyperactive or hypersensitive bladder dysfunction. J Urol. 1997;157:585–9.
41. Payne CK, Mosbaugh PG, Forrest JB, Evans RJ, Whitmore KE, Antoci JP, et al. Intravesical resiniferatoxin for the treatment of interstitial cystitis: a randomized, double-blind, placebo controlled trial. J Urol. 2005;173(5):1590–4.
42. Ham BK, Kim JH, Oh MM, Lee JG, Bae JH. Effects of combination treatment of intravesical resiniferatoxin instillation and hydrodistention in patients with refractory painful bladder syndrome/interstitial cystitis: a pilot study. Int Neurourol J. 2012;16(1):41–6.
43. Peng CH, Kuo HC. Multiple intravesical instillations of low-dose resiniferatoxin in the treatment of refractory interstitial cystitis. Urol Int. 2007;78(1):78–81.
44. Lee WC, Chuang YC, Lee WC, Chiang PH. Safety and dose flexibility clinical evaluation of intravesical liposome in patients with interstitial cystitis or painful bladder syndrome. Kaohsiung J Med Sci. 2011;27(10):437–40.
45. Fraser MO, Chuang YC, Tyagi P, Yokoyama T, Yoshimura N, Huang L, et al. Intravesical liposome administration--a novel treatment for hyperactive bladder in the rat. Urology. 2003;61(3):656–63.

21 Botulinum Toxin in Treatment of Bladder Pain Syndrome/ Interstitial Cystitis

Paulo Dinis

21.1 What Did We Get Right?

Botulinum toxin (BonTA) exerts its main therapeutic by inhibiting neuro-mediator exocytosis [1]. This was originally seen with acetylcholine hence the first diseases to be treated with BonTA injections where ocular strabismus and other striated muscular conditions [2]. In urologic diseases use of BonTA also started with application to striated muscle. In this case the urethral sphincter was targetd for treatment of sphincter-detrusor dissynergia in spinal cord injury patients [3]. With the rationale of smooth muscle relaxation, intra-vesical injections where approved initially for neurogenic detrusor over activity and later for the idiopathic overactive bladder syndrome. These applications showed great success and presently are mainstays of neurogenic and idiopathic bladder over activity treatment [4–6]. Since both the toxic effects as well as therapeutic effects of BonTA were seen as an efferent neuronal effect it was initially overlooked in the treatment of bladder pain.

P. Dinis
Department of Urology, Faculty of Medicine, Hospital de São João, Porto, Portugal
e-mail: paulodinisoliveira@gmail.com

21.2 Where Were We Off Base?

From the verification that botulinum toxin also affected sensory nerve function it was a matter of time until its use was attempted in Bladder Pain Syndrome/Interstitial Cystitis (BPS/IC). Indeed, the toxin also hinders exocytosis of sensory nerve neuro-mediators and decreases expression of fundamental receptors in nerve fiber activation such as transient receptor potential receptor vanilloid type 1 (TRPV1) and purinergic receptor type 2X3 (P2X3) [7, 8]. The fact that treatment of spastic muscle ameliorated pain by more than simple muscle relaxation turned attention to these basic science findings. Previous experience with BonTA intravesical injection in bladder overactivity showed the technique's safety and efficacy thus paving the way for trials in BPS/IC.

21.3 What Seminal Publications Changed Our Thinking?

In 2004 Smith et al., published the first results with bladder wall and trigonal injection in 13 patients with bladder pain syndrome (BPS/IC). The authors reported improvement of pain in 69% of patients [9]. Other groups soon published their results. In a pilot study, Giannantoni et al. injected 200 units (UI), sub-urothelial BonTA, to

P.M. Hanno et al. (eds.), *Bladder Pain Syndrome – An Evolution*,
https://doi.org/10.1007/978-3-319-61449-6_21

trigone and bladder floor of 14 patients. Of these, 12 patients (85.7%) showed improvement in frequency, nocturia, pain (VAS) score and increased cystometric capacity [10]. The same group reported on a prospective follow-up of 13 patients with repeat injections for 2 years. All patients received multiple site bladder wall injections totaling 200 U. A total of 58 injections were administered with a mean of 4.8 ± 0.8 injections per patient. The mean interval between two consecutive injections was 5.25 ± 0.75 months. At 1 and 4 months follow up ten patients reported a subjective improvement. Treatment efficacy was maintained in all patients during the observation period [11].

Injection technique varies among groups. Based on a previous study showing a predominance of sensory afferent distribution at the trigone [12], Pinto et al. performed injection at ten trigonal sites only with a total of 100 UI of BoNT-A, in 26 patients with refractory BPS/IC. Pain, frequency and nocturia, O'Leary-Sant Interstitial Cystitis Symptom Index (ICSI) and quality of life of all patients improved significantly. Maximal cystometric capacity also increased and the efficacy remained in >50% of the patients for 9 months [13].

In a single center, prospective randomized study, Kuo et al. injected 100 or 200 UI in 40 sites in the posterior and lateral bladder wall, combined with hydrodistension in 29 patients while 13 control patients also with BPS/IC, underwent hydrodistension only. Seventy one percent of patients in the treatment arm still showed improvement at 6 months, 55% at 12 months, and 30% at 24 months [14].

In a multicenter, randomized, double-blind, placebo controlled trial in patients with IC/BPS refractory to conventional treatment, by Kuo et al., patients were randomized to hydrodistention plus suburothelial injections of BoNT-A 100 U (BonTA group) or normal saline (control group). A total of 60 patients (8 males, 52 females) including 40 in the BonTA and 20 in the control group were enrolled. At week 8, a significantly greater reduction of pain was observed in the BonTA group. Cystometric bladder capacity also increased significantly. Success rate was 63% in the BonTA group versus 15% in the control group. Adverse events (AE) did not differ between groups [15].

A single-center, prospective, open labeled, randomized comparative study by Akiyama et al. studied BonTA application in BPS/IC patients refractory to previous hidrodistension and Hunner lesion ressection when present, performed on average for 2.7 times per patient. Patients were randomly divided into two groups: immediate injection (group A) or 1-month delayed injection (group B) of BonTA. A total of 34 patients (group A n = 18, group B n = 16) were allocated. The response rate was significantly higher in group A than group B (72.2% vs. 25.0%). When both groups were combined as a single cohort, the response rate was 73.5% at 1 month, 58.8% at 3 months, 38.2% at 6 months and 20.6% at 12 months. The mean duration of response was 5.4 months [16].

Studies generally report a limited time of the therapeutic effect spanning from *circa* 5 to 9 months, implying the need for repeat injections. However, these have been proven as effective as the initial treatment by several groups [11, 14, 17].

Adverse events (AE) were mild and infrequent in all studies and most frequently consisted of dysuria and urinary infection [11, 14, 17]. Acute urinary retention was not found in trigone-only injection studies [17, 18] and was rare in other studies [19, 20]. However no randomized head to head trials comparing bladder wall versus trigonal-only injection for BPS/IC treatment been reported either assessing efficacy or AE. In a comparative study of 72 BPS/IC patients with 89 OAB patients, both groups were treated with 100 UI of botulinum toxin applied to the bladder wall and AE were compared. Fifty eight percent of OAB patients reported at least one adverse event, including gross hematuria (9.7%), urinary tract infection (UTI) (27.8%), straining to void (8.3%), large post void residual (PVR) (31.9%) and acute urinary retention (AUR) (1.4%). On the other hand, 42.7% of BPS/IC patients found at least one AE, including UTI (6.7%), straining to void (30.3%) and large PVR (6.7%). There was neither gross hematuria nor acute urinary retention experienced in the BPS/IC patient group. Overall incidence of AEs was significantly lower in the BPS/ IC than in the OAB group. Different pathophysiological mechanisms at play in BPS/ IC and OAB might explain different AE rates for an identical treatment [21].

In the work by Akiyama et al., a total of 10 of 34 (29.4%) patients complained of voiding difficulty after treatment. Three patients (0.9%) had elevated post void residual (PVR) for the first 2 months, which resolved spontaneously. Other adverse events included transient gross hematuria (n = 1–0.3%), which also resolved spontaneously and afebrile urinary tract infection (UTI) (n = 2–0.6%).

Two meta-analyses on the use of BonTA in BPS/IC have been published. The first evidence-based meta-analysis investigated efficacy and safety data from five randomized controlled studies including a total of 252 subjects (133 in experimental and 119 in control groups).This study showed that subjective indexes such as VAS and O'Leary Sant scores were significantly improved following BoNTA treatment compared to placebo. Although there was no significant difference between treated and control patients, except for dysuria (31%), AEs did include urinary retention (6%), UTI (6%), large post void residual (8.3%) and hematuria (3.6%) [19]. Another meta-analysis comprising 183 active treatment patients and 134 control patients reported similar findings, in efficacy and safety parameters [20].

21.4 Where Do We Go from Here?

Despite the obvious success obtained with BonTA its application in BPS/IC will benefit from better phenotyping of BPS/IC patients. Basic and epidemiological studies as well as individual clinical manifestations clearly indicate that BPS/IC encompasses more than one disease. A clearer understanding of this will increase the strength of indications for treatment with BonTA. Of course neither BonTA is an optimal molecule nor is intravesical bladder wall injection the most desirable technique to apply it. For the treatment of pain *per se* an ideal drug to be used in a similar approach as BonTA would have specificity for sensory afferent nerve fibers. This would in effect abrogate the most frequent (voiding difficulty) and the most dreaded AE—urinary retention. On the other hand the need to inject the bladder increases morbidity of the procedure due to possible induction of pain, infection and hematuria. Bladder instillation of BonTA is being investigated. Simultaneous administration of BonTA with drugs to denude urothelium, thermosensitive hidrogels or encapsulated in lipossomes to enable its uptake into the bladder wall are some possible options and already show potential efficacy in human pilot studies. Possible circumscription of BonTA effect to sensory fibers was reported in one study with lipossome encapsulated toxin [22]. Physical means are also being explored for intravesical delivery of BonTA namely iontophoresis and shockwave use [23–25].

Since its first application in Urology, BonTA intravesical injection has progressively been proven as effective and safe for the treatment of BPS/IC. It is presently recommended by both American and European guidelines before more invasive surgical treatments [26, 27]. However BonTA application in BPS/IC still warrants a delivery technique with less invasiveness and a better targeted therapeutical effect.

References

1. Schiavo G, Rossetto O, Benfenati F, Poulain B, Montecucco C. Tetanus and botulinum neurotoxins are zinc proteases specific for components of the neuroexocytosis apparatus. Ann N Y Acad Sci. 1994;710:65–75.
2. Scott AB. Botulinum toxin injection into extraocular muscles as an alternative to strabismus surgery. J Pediatr Ophthalmol Strabismus. 1980;17(1):21–5.
3. Dykstra DD, Sidi AA, Scott AB, Pagel JM, Goldish GD. Effects of botulinum A toxin on detrusor-sphincter dyssynergia in spinal cord injury patients. J Urol. 1988;139(5):919–22.
4. Schurch B, Stohrer M, Kramer G, Schmid DM, Gaul G, Hauri D. Botulinum-A toxin for treating detrusor hyperreflexia in spinal cord injured patients: a new alternative to anticholinergic drugs? Preliminary results. J Urol. 2000;164(3 Pt 1):692–7.
5. Sahai A, Khan MS, Dasgupta P. Efficacy of botulinum toxin-A for treating idiopathic detrusor overactivity: results from a single center, randomized, double-blind, placebo controlled trial. J Urol. 2007;177(6):2231–6.

6. Flynn MK, Webster GD, Amundsen CL. The effect of botulinum-A toxin on patients with severe urge urinary incontinence. J Urol. 2004;172(6 Pt 1):2316–20.
7. Welch MJ, Purkiss JR, Foster KA. Sensitivity of embryonic rat dorsal root ganglia neurons to Clostridium botulinum neurotoxins. Toxicon. 2000;38(2):245–58.
8. Apostolidis A, Popat R, Yiangou Y, Cockayne D, Ford AP, Davis JB, et al. Decreased sensory receptors P2X3 and TRPV1 in suburothelial nerve fibers following intradetrusor injections of botulinum toxin for human detrusor overactivity. J Urol. 2005;174(3):977–82. discussion 82-3
9. Smith CP, Radziszewski P, Borkowski A, Somogyi GT, Boone TB, Chancellor MB. Botulinum toxin a has antinociceptive effects in treating interstitial cystitis. Urology. 2004;64(5):871–5. discussion 5
10. Giannantoni A, Costantini E, Di Stasi SM, Tascini MC, Bini V, Porena M. Botulinum A toxin intravesical injections in the treatment of painful bladder syndrome: a pilot study. Eur Urol. 2006;49(4):704–9.
11. Giannantoni A, Mearini E, Del Zingaro M, Proietti S, Porena M. Two-year efficacy and safety of botulinum a toxin intravesical injections in patients affected by refractory painful bladder syndrome. Curr Drug Deliv. 2010;7(1):1–4.
12. Avelino A, Cruz C, Nagy I, Cruz F. Vanilloid receptor 1 expression in the rat urinary tract. Neuroscience. 2002;109(4):787–98.
13. Pinto R, Lopes T, Frias B, Silva A, Silva JA, Silva CM, et al. Trigonal injection of botulinum toxin A in patients with refractory bladder pain syndrome/interstitial cystitis. Eur Urol. 2010;58(3):360–5.
14. Kuo HC, Chancellor MB. Comparison of intravesical botulinum toxin type A injections plus hydrodistention with hydrodistention alone for the treatment of refractory interstitial cystitis/painful bladder syndrome. BJU Int. 2009;104(5):657–61.
15. Kuo HC, Jiang YH, Tsai YC, Kuo YC. Intravesical botulinum toxin-A injections reduce bladder pain of interstitial cystitis/bladder pain syndrome refractory to conventional treatment - A prospective, multicenter, randomized, double-blind, placebo-controlled clinical trial. Neurourol Urodyn. 2016;35(5):609–14.
16. Akiyama Y, Nomiya A, Niimi A, Yamada Y, Fujimura T, Nakagawa T, et al. Botulinum toxin type A injection for refractory interstitial cystitis: a randomized comparative study and predictors of treatment response. Int J Urol. 2015;22(9):835–41.
17. Pinto R, Lopes T, Silva J, Silva C, Dinis P, Cruz F. Persistent therapeutic effect of repeated injections of onabotulinum toxin a in refractory bladder pain syndrome/interstitial cystitis. J Urol. 2013;189(2):548–53.
18. Kasyan G, Pushkar D. 822 randomized controlled trial for efficacy of botulinum toxin type a in treatment of patients suffering bladder pain syndrome/interstitial cystitis with hunners' lesions preliminary results. J Urol. 2012;187(4):e335–e6.
19. Shim SR, Cho YJ, Shin IS, Kim JH. Efficacy and safety of botulinum toxin injection for interstitial cystitis/bladder pain syndrome: a systematic review and meta-analysis. Int Urol Nephrol. 2016;48(8):1215–27.
20. Wang J, Wang Q, Wu Q, Chen Y, Wu P. Intravesical botulinum toxin A injections for bladder pain syndrome/interstitial cystitis: a systematic review and meta-analysis of controlled studies. Med Sci Monit. 2016;22:3257–67.
21. Kuo YC, Kuo HC. Adverse events of intravesical onabotulinumtoxinA injection between patients with overactive bladder and interstitial cystitis--different mechanisms of action of botox on bladder dysfunction? Toxins (Basel). 2016;8(3):75.
22. Kuo HC, Liu HT, Chuang YC, Birder LA, Chancellor MB. Pilot study of liposome-encapsulated onabotulinumtoxina for patients with overactive bladder: a single-center study. Eur Urol. 2014;65(6):1117–24.
23. Ahmadi H, Montaser-Kouhsari L, Kajbafzadeh A-M. 744 intravesical electromotive botulinum toxin type A administration: preliminary findings for the treatment of children with myelomeningocele and refractory neurogenic detrusor overactivity. J Urol. 2010;183(4):e291.
24. Stav K, Vinshtok Y, Jeshurun M, Ivgy-May N, Gerassi T, Zisman A. PD20-03 pilot study evaluating safety and feasibility of intravesical instillation of botulinum toxin in hydrogel-based slow release delivery system in PBS/IC patients. J Urol. 2015;193(4):e398.
25. Tyagi P, Kashyap M, Yoshimura N, Chancellor M, Chermansky CJ. Past, present and future of chemodenervation with botulinum toxin in the treatment of overactive bladder. J Urol. 2017;197(4):982–90.
26. Hanno PM, Erickson D, Moldwin R, Faraday MM, American Urological A. Diagnosis and treatment of interstitial cystitis/bladder pain syndrome: AUA guideline amendment. J Urol. 2015;193(5):1545–53.
27. Engeler D, Baranowski AP, Borovicka J, Dinis-Oliveira P, Elneil S, Hughes J, et al. EAU guidelines on chronic pelvic pain. Arnhem: EAU Guidelines Office; 2016.

Intravesical Therapy and Its Evolution Over Three Decades, A European View

22

Mauro Cervigni

22.1 What Did We Get Right?

The finding of an effective and specific therapy for IC/BPS remains a challenge because of the lack of a consensus regarding the causes and the inherent difficulties in the diagnosis. One of the last recent hypothesis is that IC/BPS could be pathophysiologically related to a disruption of the bladder mucosa surface layer with consequent loss of glycosaminoglycans (GAGs). This class of mucopolysaccharides has hydrorepellent properties and their alteration expose the urothelium to many urinary toxic agents (GAGs). The urothelium consist of three layers of cells [1–3] (basal, intermediate and apical or umbrella cells) This outer layer comprises the main impermeable and protective barrier against urine. The barrier function is comprised also of other defensive mechanism such as: tight junctions, uroplakin and a dense layer of glycosaminoglycan (GAG) on the apical surface. The removal of GAG layer causes loss of the apical cells within 24 h and leads to enhanced permeability. When these substances penetrate the bladder wall a chain is triggered in the submucosa. Here nerve terminals produce inflammatory mediators causing mast cell degranulation and histamine secretion with consequent vasodilatation and inflammatory exudate. The consequence of this inflammatory response is the stimulation of C fibers with mast cell activation and histamine release. This produce consequent bladder pain and release of neuropetides with a consequent damage to the mucosa and fibrosis of the submucosa [4–6].

Restoring the GAG with exogenous GAG restores impermeability to baseline levels [7] and also substantially inhibits the recruitment of inflammatory cells to permeabilized areas [8].

The major classes of GAG include hyaluronic acid (HA), heparin sulphate, heparin, chondroitin 4-sulphate, chondroitin 6-sulphate, dermatan sulphate and keratan sulphate [9]. In order to improve the integrity and function of the bladder lining, GAG layer replenishment therapy is widely accepted as therapy for patients with IC/BPS who have poor or inadequate response to conventional therapy [10]. Currently, chondroitin sulfate (CS), heparin, HA, and pentosan polysulfate (PPS), and combinations of two GAGs (CS and HA) are the available substances with different effectiveness rates in patients with IC/BPS.

Four different products are commercially available for GAG replenishment including CS, heparin, HA and PPS. Each product has different concentrations and dosage formulations. Recently, a combination of CS and HA is the latest commercially available product.

M. Cervigni
Interstitial Cystitis Referral Center and Female Pelvic Medicine and Reconstructive Surgery Center, Foundation University Hospital A. Gemelli, Catholic University, Rome, Italy
e-mail: mauro.cervigni@policlinicogemelli.it

P.M. Hanno et al. (eds.), *Bladder Pain Syndrome – An Evolution*,
https://doi.org/10.1007/978-3-319-61449-6_22

22.2 Where Were We Off Base?

22.2.1 Sodium Pentosan Polysulfate (PPS)

PPS is a semi-synthetic, sulfated polysaccharide, which is chemically and structurally similar to heparin and GAG. A proposed mechanism is that the drug replaces the damaged parts of the GAG layer that lines the bladder [11]. It has been reported that PPS reduces bladder permeability based on the potassium sensitivity test [12]. Currently, PPS is the only oral therapy approved by the FDA for IC/PBS [13].

However, randomized controlled trials (RCTs) have shown mixed results in its efficacy. Mulholland and Parsons separately reported significantly improved pain and urgency symptoms from baseline at 3-month follow-up [14, 15]. La Rock and Sant [16] suggested that in comparison with oral therapy, intravesical sodium pentosan polysulphate (SPP) therapy promotes direct absorption of the drug by the bladder. Conversely, Holm-Bentzen et al. failed to demonstrate any difference at 4-month follow-up compared to placebo [17]. Increasing treatment doses does not appear to improve efficacy from the 100 mg 3 times a day (TID) dosing. Diarrhea, abdominal pain, and rectal bleeding are the most common side effects and have been found to be dose-related. Alopecia was also noted in 5% of patients in one study [18]. High-quality evidence demonstrates mixed support for this therapy. Therefore, given the moderate side effect profile, PPS is recommended as a second-line therapy for IC/PBS [19].

22.2.2 Hyaluronic Acid (HA)

Intravesical HA was the first GAG substance used for IC/PBS. Morales et al. published the first study in 1996; they found a complete or partial response rate of 71% for up to 1 year [20]. In patients with IC/BPS, the concentration of this acid is decreased and urothelial permeability toward potassium compounds is increased, causing an increase in bladder pain. HA inhibits leukocyte chemotactic and phagocytic functions, and reduces the permeability of the synovial membrane [21]. HA acts on urothelial cells in three distinct ways: by increasing secretion of GAG enzymes; this leads to increased GAG secretion, leading to restored homoeostasis and eventual normal GAG barrier production. HA through a direct physicochemical interaction with the cells' surface decreases the permeability of the urothelium. HA acts on the third pathway by decreasing secretion of pro-inflammatory cytokines IL-6 and IL-8 from the urothelial cells, decreasing immune cell infiltration to the urothelium and decreasing inflammation [22]. HA has been the subject of multiple studies and has shown a wide range of symptom improvement, from 30 to 85% [23–25]. In 2011 Engelhardt and his collaborators reported their long-term results of intravesical HA therapy; they observed a 50% complete bladder symptom remission at the 5-year follow-up without any additional therapy, while 41.7% with symptom recurrence improved with HA maintenance therapy [26]. Not all the studies have shown a significant effect of HA. For example in a double-blind, placebo-controlled, multicentre clinical study with this GAG in different preparations (40 or 200 mg/cc), no significant efficacy of sodium hyaluronate compared to placebo was found for interstitial cystitis (IC) patients. However, further details, including patient selection, inclusion/exclusion criteria, definition of improvement/success, are not available [27]. In the study of Daha et al. hydrodistention in combination with HA with potassium chloride (KCl), in addition to sodium chloride (NaCl), were used as a treatment of IC/BPS. With the combined use of KCl and NaCl, pain was improved by 62.5% and 71.48% respectively [28]. HA does not provide immediate relief of symptoms, as some time is required before the onset of regeneration of the GAG layer. By contrast, lidocaine (a local anesthetic) can reduce sensory ending excitability in the bladder and help with the control and immediate relief of pain and voiding frequency. For this reason, Lv proposed a combined therapy that may lead to an immediate relief of symptoms by addicting lidocaine to HA. With this treatment, voiding frequency was reduced by 67.25% and pain was reduced by 70.82% [29].

22.2.3 Chondroitin Sulfate (CS)

CS is another natural proteoglycan present in the GAG layer of the bladder epithelium. Like HA, intravesical instillation of this molecule has been proposed as a treatment for patients with IC/BPS, to promote regeneration of GAG in the bladder urothelium. Results from a recent experiment revealed good control of urinary symptoms and pain, suggesting that the use of this drug in IC/BPS may be of benefit. Intravesical CS therapy efficiency was evaluated by Steinhoff and colleagues in an open-label 12-month study. In this study, the authors treated 18 patients with 40-mL instillations of CS 0.2% weekly for 4 weeks and then monthly for 12 months. They found a response rate for symptom improvement of 67% [30]. In an uncontrolled open multicenter study of 53 IC patients, instillations of CS 2% produced a 60% response rate at 6 months [31]. In contrast, a recently published RCT failed to show superiority of CS 2.0% over control after 6 weeks of treatment. In that study, most patients reported a clinical benefit, but the difference between treatment and control group was not statistically significant [32]. According to the 2012 data of the Brazilian Ministry of Health, the production of intravesical HA was stimulated by instillation of CS; a substance that blocks the action of lytic enzymes and stimulates proteoglycan synthesis by inducing increased HA levels, thus reconstituting the urothelium. Nickel et al. conducted an interventional study by using bladder hydrodistention with 20 mL of saline associated with 2% CS, and found an improvement in pain and urinary urgency of 47% and a decrease in voiding frequency by 51.8% [33].

22.3 What Seminal Publications Changed Our Thinking?

22.3.1 CS and HA

A combination of two GAG containing CS (2.0%) and low molecular weight HA (1.6%) is the latest available substance for the GAG replenishment therapy.

In an open-label single arm study by Porru and colleagues, the efficiency of intravesical CS/HA combination therapy was evaluated in IC/PBS patients. Twenty-two patients with IC/BPS received intravesical instillations (40 mL) of sodium HA 1.6% and CS 2.0% in 0.9% saline solution (IALURIL®) (IBSA, Lugano, Switzerland) once weekly for 8 weeks, then once every 2 weeks for the next 6 months. Parameters included visual analogue scale (VAS) for pain and urgency, number of void per day, mean voiding volume, Interstitial Cystitis Symptom Index (ICSI) and Pain Urgency Frequency (PUF) questionnaire. The score for urgency was reduced from 6.5 to 3.6 ($P = 0.0001$), with a reduction in pain scores from an average of 5.6 to 3.2 ($P = 0.0001$). The average urine volume increased from 129.7 to 162 mL ($P < 0.0001$), with a reduction in the number of voids in 24 hours, from 14 to 11.6 ($P < 0.0001$). The IC Symptom and Problem Index decreased from 25.7 to 20.3 ($P < 0.0001$), and the PUF score, from 18.7 to 12.8 ($P < 0.0001$) [34]. Cervigni and colleagues reported the long-term results of intravesical CS/HA therapy in 12 IC/BPS patients refractory to other treatments. They used a combination of HA 1.6% and CS 2.0% over a period of 3 years assessing symptoms and quality of life using a visual analogue scale, 3-day voiding diaries and validated questionnaires. Improvements in bladder function were sustained for 3 years (mean number of daily voids decreased from 17.8 at baseline to 15.5 at 9 months and 11.9 at 3 years, and mean volume per void from 136.8 mL at baseline to 143.9 mL at 9 months and 180.9 mL at 3 years). Quality of life assessments confirmed these improvements [35]. Ömer Gülpınarite studied 53 BPS IC patients with inadequate clinical response after 6 months of conservative treatment comparing for the first time intravesical HA/CS combination and intravesical HA. In total, 53 patients met the study criteria. There were 30 patients in the HA-CS group (mean age: 48.47 years old) and 23 patients in the HA group (mean age: 49.61 years old) ($P > 0.05$). The initial PST was positive in 71.7% patients (38/53) overall with no difference between groups ($P > 0.05$). Responses for VAS, ICSI, Interstitial Cystitis Problem Index (ICPI), 24-hour frequency/nocturia statistically improved in both groups at 6 months. There was no significant difference in symptomatic improvement ($P > 0.05$). Eight patients had mild adverse events [36].

More recently Cervigni et al. [37] published a randomized open-label multicenter study comparing the efficacy, safety, and costs of of Intravesical instillation of hyaluronic acid (HA) plus chondroitin sulfate (CS) (Ialuril®, IBSA) versus dimethyl sulfoxide in women with BPS/IC in 110 women. The allocation ratio (HA/CS:DMSO) was 2:1. Thirteen weekly instillations of HA (1.6%)/CS (2.0%) or 50% DMSO were given. Patients were evaluated at 3 (end-of-treatment) and 6 months. Primary endpoint was reduction in pain intensity at 6 months by visual analogue scale (VAS) versus baseline. Secondary efficacy measurements were quality of life and economic analyses. A significant reduction in pain intensity was observed at 6 months in both treatment groups versus baseline ($P < 0.0001$) in the intention-to-treat population. Treatment with HA/CS resulted in a greater reduction in pain intensity at 6 months compared with DMSO for the per-protocol population (mean VAS reduction 44.77 ± 25.07 vs. 28.89 ± 31.14, respectively; $P = 0.0186$). There were no significant differences between treatment groups in secondary outcomes. At least one adverse event was reported in 14.86% and 30.56% of patients in the HA/CS and DMSO groups, respectively. There were significantly fewer treatment-related adverse events for HA/CS versus DMSO (1.35% vs. 22.22%; $P = 0.001$). Considering direct healthcare costs, the incremental cost-effectiveness ratio of HA/CS versus DMSO fell between 3735€/quality-adjusted life years (QALY) and 8003€/QALY. Treatment with HA/CS appears to be as effective as DMSO with a potentially more favorable safety profile. Both treatments increased health-related quality of life, while HA/CS showed a more acceptable cost-effectiveness profile.

22.4 Where Do We Go from Here?

IC/BPS remains a prevalent, but untreated disease with a poorly understood pathophysiology. Nonetheless, research suggests that (I) disruption of the bladder GAG/ proteoglycan layer, (II) upregulated immune/inflammatory response, (III) neural upregulation, and (IV) pelvic floor dysfunction may all play a role in the pathophysiology of the disease.

HA and HA/CS therapy are effective treatment options for patients with IC/BPS who had inadequate response to conservative treatment, in the short term. Obviously this treatment must be plugged into a multimodal protocol of associated and combined therapies.

Further randomized controlled studies with a larger number of patients and a longer follow-up period are needed to confirm these encouraging results and to optimize the treatment protocol for a sustained long-term therapeutic effect.

Recently there is an increasing interest in the use of liposomes as carriers for drugs administered by the intravesical route. The lipidic bilayer structure of liposomes facilitates their adherence to the apical membrane surface of luminal cells in the bladder, and their vesicular shape allows them to co-opt the endocytosis for bladder uptake after instillation [38].

References

1. Hicks RM, Ketterer B, Warren RC. The ultrastructure and chemistry of the luminal plasma membrane of the mammalian urinary bladder: a structure with low permeability to water and ions. Philos Trans R Soc Lond Ser B Biol Sci. 1974;268:23–38.
2. Congiu T, Radice R, Raspanti M, et al. The 3D structure of the human urinary bladder mucosa: a scanning electron microscopy study. J Submicrosc Cytol Pathol. 2004;36:45–53.
3. Jost SP, Gosling JA, Dixon JS. The morphology of normal human bladder urothelium. J Anat. 1989;167:103–15.
4. Bassi P, Costantini E, Foley S, et al. Glycosaminoglycan therapy for bladder diseases: emerging new treatments. Eur Urol. 2011;10:451–9.
5. Iavazzo C, Athanasiou S, Pitsouni E, et al. Hyaluronic acid: an effective alternative treatment of interstitial cystitis, recurrent urinary tract infections, and hemorrhagic cystitis? Eur Urol. 2007;51:1534–40. discussion 1540-1
6. Parsons CL. Prostatitis, interstitial cystitis, chronic pelvic pain, and urethral syndrome share a common pathophysiology: lower urinary dysfunctional epithelium and potassium recycling. Urology. 2003;62:976–82.
7. Hauser PJ, Buethe DA, Califano J, et al. Restoring barrier function to acid damaged bladder by intravesical chondroitin sulfate. J Urol. 2009;182:2477–82.
8. Engles CD, Hauser PJ, Abdullah SN, et al. Intravesical chondroitin sulfate inhibits recruitment of inflamma-

tory cells in an acute acid damage "leaky bladder" model of cystitis. Urology. 2012;79:483.e13–7.
9. Hurst RE. Structure, function, and pathology of proteoglycans and glycosaminoglycans in the urinary tract. World J Urol. 1994;12:3–10.
10. Fall M, Baranowski AP, Elneil S, et al. EAU guidelines on chronic pelvic pain. Eur Urol. 2010;57:35–48.
11. Parsons CL. The therapeutic role of sulfated polysaccharides in the urinary bladder. Urol Clin North Am. 1994;21:93–100.
12. Parsons CL, Forrest J, Nickel JC, et al. Effect of pentosan polysulfate therapy on intravesical potassium sensitivity. Urology. 2002;59:329–33.
13. Davis EL, El Khoudary SR, Talbott EO, et al. Safety and efficacy of the use of intravesical and oral pentosan polysulfate sodium for interstitial cystitis: a randomized double-blind clinical trial. J Urol. 2008;179:177–85.
14. Mulholland SG, Hanno P, Parsons CL, et al. Pentosan polysulfate sodium for therapy of interstitial cystitis. A double-blind placebo-controlled clinical study. Urology. 1990;35:552–8.
15. Parsons CL, Benson G, Childs SJ, et al. A quantitatively controlled method to study prospectively interstitial cystitis and demonstrate the efficacy of pentosanpolysulfate. J Urol. 1993;150:845–8.
16. La Rock DR, Sant GR. Intravesical therapies for interstitial cystitis. In: Sant GR, editor. Interstitial cystitis. Philadelphia, PA: Lippincott-Raven; 1997.
17. Holm-Bentzen M, Jacobsen F, Nerstrøm B, et al. A prospective double-blind clinically controlled multicenter trial of sodium pentosanpolysulfate in the treatment of interstitial cystitis and related painful bladder disease. J Urol. 1987;138:503–7.
18. Nickel JC, Barkin J, Forrest J, et al. Randomized, double-blind, dose-ranging study of pentosan polysulfate sodium for interstitial cystitis. Urology. 2005;65:654–8.
19. Hanno PM, Burks DA, Clemens JQ, et al. AUA guideline for the diagnosis and treatment of interstitial cystitis/ bladder pain syndrome. J Urol. 2011;185:2162–70.
20. Morales A, Emerson L, Nickel JC, et al. Intravesical hyaluronic acid in the treatment of refractory interstitial cystitis. J Urol. 1996;156:45–8.
21. Parsons CL, Lilly JD, Stein P. Epithelial dysfunction in nonbacterial cystitis (interstitial cystitis). J Urol. 1991;145:732–5.
22. Rooney P, Srivastava A, Watson L, et al. Hyaluronic acid decreases IL-6 and IL-8 secretion and permeability in an inflammatory model of interstitial cystitis. Acta Biomater. 2015;19:66–75.
23. Gupta SK, Pidcock L, Parr NJ. The potassium sensitivity test: a predictor of treatment response in interstitial cystitis. BJU Int. 2005;96:1063–6.
24. Kallestrup EB, Jorgensen SS, Nordling J, et al. Treatment of interstitial cystitis with Cystistat: a hyaluronic acid product. Scand J Urol Nephrol. 2005;39:143–7.
25. Riedl CR, Engelhardt PF, Daha KL, et al. Hyaluronan treatment of interstitial cystitis/painful bladder syndrome. Int Urogynecol J Pelvic Floor Dysfunct. 2008;19:717–21.
26. Engelhardt PF, Morakis N, Daha LK, et al. Long-term results of intravesical hyaluronan therapy in bladder pain syndrome/interstitial cystitis. Int Urogynecol J. 2011;22:401–5.
27. Hanno P, Baranowski A, Fall M, et al. Painful bladder syndrome (including interstitial cystitis). In: Abrams PH, Wein AJ, Cardozo L, et al., editors. Incontinence. 3rd ed. Paris: Health Publications Limited; 2005. p. 1456–520.
28. Daha LK, Riedl CR, Lazar D, et al. Do cystometric findings predict the results of intravesical hyaluronic acid in women with interstitial cystitis? Eur Urol. 2005;47:393–7.
29. Lv YS, Zhou HL, Mao HP, et al. Intravesical hyaluronic acid and alkalinized lidocaine for the treatment of severe painful bladder syndrome/interstitial cystitis. Int Urogynecol J. 2012;23:1715–20.
30. Steinhoff G, Ittah B, Rowan S. The efficacy of chondroitin sulfate 0.2% in treating interstitial cystitis. Can J Urol. 2002;9:1454–8.
31. Nickel JC, Egerdie B, Downey J, et al. A real-life multicentre clinical practice study to evaluate the efficacy and safety of intravesical chondroitin sulphate for the treatment of interstitial cystitis. BJU Int. 2009;103:56–60.
32. Nickel JC, Egerdie RB, Steinhoff G, et al. A multicenter, randomized, double-blind, parallel group pilot evaluation of the efficacy and safety of intravesical sodium chondroitin sulfate versus vehicle control in patients with interstitial cystitis/painful bladder syndrome. Urology. 2010;76:804–9.
33. Nickel JC, Hanno P, Kumar K, et al. Second multicenter, randomized, double-blind, parallel-group evaluation of effectiveness and safety of intravesical sodium chondroitin sulfate compared with inactive vehicle control in subjects with interstitial cystitis/ bladder pain syndrome. Urology. 2012;79:1220–4.
34. Porru D, Leva F, Parmigiani A, et al. Impact of intravesical hyaluronic acid and chondroitin sulfate on bladder pain syndrome/interstitial cystitis. Int Urogynecol J. 2012;23:1193–9.
35. Cervigni M, Natale F, Nasta L, et al. Intravesical hyaluronic acid and chondroitin sulphate for bladder pain syndrome/interstitial cystitis: long-term treatment results. Int Urogynecol J. 2012;23:1187–92.
36. Gülpınar O, Kayış A, Süer E, et al. Clinical comparision of intravesical hyaluronic acid and hyaluronic acid-chondroitin sulphate therapy for patients with bladder pain syndrome/interstitital cystitis. Can Urol Assoc J. 2014;8:E610–4.
37. Cervigni M, Sommariva M, Tenaglia R, et al. A randomized, open-label, multicenter study of the efficacy and safety of intravesical hyaluronic acid and chondroitin sulfate versus dimethyl sulfoxide in women with bladder pain syndrome/interstitial cystitis. Neurourol Urodyn. 2017;36(4):1178–86.
38. Tyagi P, Kashyap M, Majima T, et al. Intravesical liposome therapy for interstitial cystitis. Int J Urol. 2017;24(4):262–71.

23 The Use of Heparin

Arndt van Ophoven

23.1 Where Were We Off Base?

From its first introduction as a therapeutic agent for IC in 1963 on treatment results of heparin use have been rarely but constantly reported until today. The preferred route of administration is by intravesical instillation although patients suffering from bladder pain syndrome often fear and wish to avoid repetitive catheterization. Thus, the subcutaneous route of administration as reported for the first time by Gunnar Lose in 1983 and summarized in Chap. 15, offers an alternative, less painful and minimal invasive approach. However, in contrast to subcutaneous administration which requires the monitoring of clotting parameters, no such information is required for the safe use of instillations which increases their feasibility regarding follow up monitoring of patients and has added to their preference as a mode of administration.

23.2 What Did We Get Right?

The use of heparin in the treatment of bladder pain syndromes is unchanged based on the hypothesis that the glycosaminoglycan-rich bladder surface mucus is the primary regulator of epithelial permeability and that a structurally similar exogenous sulfated polysaccharide such as heparin could effectively treat the painful bladder by compensating for the dysfunction of natural bladder mucus. Heparin is believed to work by replacing or aiding in the recovery of the individual's dysfunctional bladder mucus, subsequently reducing epithelial permeability and protecting from symptom provocation by noxious molecules.

Intravesical heparin in the management of IC/BPS has been studied in controlled and non-controlled trials enrolling more than 100 treated patients and demonstrating efficacy rates ranging from 56 to 94%. AUA guidelines recommend intravesical heparin as a second-line treatment option, having potential benefit in a subset of patients with an uncertain benefit/risk ratio. However, adverse events reported were not serious. In a controlled trial, minor events in patients receiving alkalinized lidocaine in combination with heparin were similar to placebo in frequency and type, affecting approximately 30–50% of patients and including headache, dizziness, lightheadedness, and bladder or urethral pain. No increases in activated partial thromboplastin time or prothrombin time were observed. Bladder discomfort occurred with every instillation in 60% of patients treated with intravesical heparin. In an open-label study, gross hematuria was observed only on the day of instillation and was not associated with systemic coagulation disorder.

A. van Ophoven
Division of Neuro-Urology, Marien Hospital Herne, University Hospital Ruhr-Universität Bochum, Hölkeskampring 40, 44625 Herne, Germany
e-mail: arndt.vanophoven@marienhospital-herne.de

P.M. Hanno et al. (eds.), *Bladder Pain Syndrome – An Evolution*,
https://doi.org/10.1007/978-3-319-61449-6_23

Personal experience with heparin was made during a prospective controlled study to evaluate the safety and efficacy of the combined administration of oral pentosanpolysulfate (PPS) and subcutaneous low-dose heparin, still representing the only controlled study on subcutaneous use of the agent. This trial thus partially filled the lack that "no controlled studies documenting the effect of subctaneous heparin" had been done as stated in Chap. 15 by Gunnar Lose 20 years before publication of the trial.

41 IC patients reporting efficacy of oral PPS medication were divided into a major-, intermediate-, and minor PPS response group, according to the extent of their therapeutic response to PPS. Patients received 3 × 5000 IU/d heparin for 2 days, followed by 2 × 5000 IU/d for 12 days. Maintenance dose was 5000 IU/d heparin. 17 patients randomly taking exclusively PPS served as control. In summary the subcutaneous administration of low-dose heparin appeared to be a safe and efficacious adjunct to oral PPS medication, with a cumulative effect of the two drugs predominantly observed in patients with an initial minor response to PPS. Our results supported the etiological concept of an impaired vesical glycosaminoglycan layer function as a crucial factor for the induction of IC symptoms. Since it is known that heparin profoundly inhibits mast cells our results additionally shed further light on the importance of mast cells in IC pathogenesis. We further discussed that heparin may unfold its symptom ameliorating effect by its inhibiting impact on purinergic mechanisms that are deeply involved in the neuroinflammatory processes reported for BPS/IC. Recent observations suggest that bladder purinergic mechanisms are important in bladder sensory function and are altered in BPS/IC including data that heparin attenuates stretch-activated ATP release and blocks purinergic signaling in cultured BPS/IC bladder urothelial cells.

23.3 Where Do We Go from Here?

Even 30 years after Loses book chapter on the efficacy of subctaneous heparin for the amelioration of BPS/IC, its administration, irrespective of the individually preferred route, should still be on the therapeutic landscape of any physician striving to offer more than basic medical supply to these patients. However, more clinical and scientific data to fully elucidate and explain the therapeutic potential of heparin for BPS/IC is desirable and still mandatory almost 55 years after its first use. Unfortunately, current academic and pharmaceutical research structures are compelled to focus on speedy financial or scientific return of investment and are thus prone to neglect such "old and cheap" treatment approaches.

References

1. Baykal K, Senkul T, Sen B, Karademir K, Adayener C, Erden D. Intravesical heparin and peripheral neuromodulation on interstitial cystitis. Urol Int. 2005;74(4):361–4.
2. Kuo HC. Urodynamic results of intravesical heparin therapy for women with frequency urgency syndrome and interstitial cystitis. J Formos Med Assoc. 2001;100(5):309–14.
3. Nomiya A, Naruse T, Niimi A, et al. On- and post-treatment symptom relief by repeated instillations of heparin and alkalized lidocaine in interstitial cystitis. Int J Urol. 2013;20(11):1118–22.
4. Parsons CL. Successful downregulation of bladder sensory nerves with combination of heparin and alkalinized lidocaine in patients with interstitial cystitis. Urology. 2005;65(1):45–8.
5. Parsons CL, Housley T, Schmidt JD, Lebow D. Treatment of interstitial cystitis with intravesical heparin. Br J Urol. 1994;73(5):504–7.
6. Parsons CL, Koziol JA, Proctor JG, Zupkas P, Argade S. Heparin and alkalinized lidocaine versus alkalinized lidocaine for treatment of interstitial cystitis symptoms. Can J Urol. 2015;22(2):7739–44.
7. Parsons CL, Zupkas P, Proctor J, et al. Alkalinized lidocaine and heparin provide immediate relief of pain and urgency in patients with interstitial cystitis. J Sex Med. 2012;9(1):207–12.
8. Taneja R, Jawade KK. A rational combination of intravesical and systemic agents for the treatment of interstitial cystitis. Scand J Urol Nephrol. 2007;41(6):511–5.
9. van Ophoven A, Heinecke A, Hertle L. Safety and efficacy of concurrent application of oral pentosan polysulfate and subcutaneous low-dose heparin for patients with interstitial cystitis. Urology. 2005;66(4):707–11.
10. Weaver RG, Dougherty TF, Natoli CA. Recent concepts of interstitial cystitis. J Urol. 1963;89:377–83.
11. Welk BK, Teichman JM. Dyspareunia response in patients with interstitial cystitis treated with intravesical lidocaine, bicarbonate, and heparin. Urology. 2008;71(1):67–70.

What Happened to Eosinophilic Cationic Protein: A Dead End

24

Philip Hanno

Eosinophil cationic protein (ECP) is a single cationic polypeptide chain consisting of 133 amino acids. ECP is a mediator in host immune response to parasites, bacteria and viruses. Much of the literature on this protein focuses on its role in eosinophil-related disorders like asthma. ECP correlates with airway inflammation but not airway hyper-responsiveness. It is not diagnostic of asthma but is related to severity and can be used to monitor effects of asthma treatment [1, 2]. Concentrations of ECP correlate with the clinical severity of chronic allergic conjunctival disease [3]. Although present in numerous biological fluids, sample management is complex and serum has become the main avenue of determination used in the laboratory setting. The ECP molecule participates in a large number of biological reactions, which makes it an unacceptable diagnostic marker due to low diagnostic specificity [4].

24.1 What We Got Right

The search for a biomarker for the diagnosis and phenotyping of bladder pain syndrome (BPS) has been a priority for many decades. In chapter 16 of the original text, Lose and Frandsen reviewed their work from the 1980's in which they observed an increased level of eosinophil cationic protein in the urine of patients with interstitial cystitis. Around the same time, Holm-Bentzen had demonstrated an elevated urinary excretion of metabolites of histamine in these patients. Lose and Frandsen were hopeful the urinary-ECP would provide a new tool to study patients with bladder pain syndrome and perhaps select patients with detrusor mastocytosis which at that time was considered a potential histologic confirmation of the disorder. Publications suggesting that eosinophilic infiltration of the bowel in patients with chronic bowel disease could be a marker of activity and prognosis stimulated their work.

P. Hanno
Stanford University School of Medicine,
Stanford, CA, USA
e-mail: philip.hanno@stanford.edu

24.2 What Were We Off Base

Thirty years later it appears that mast cells may not be the specific biomarker for bladder pain syndrome that was presumed. While subepithelial mast cell distribution is found to be characteristic of BPS in patients with Hunner lesions, Gamper et al. concluded that detrusor mastocytosis had poor predictive value for BPS and that mast cell assessment did not distinguish BPS without Hunner lesions from overactive bladder syndrome [5]. Submucosal mast cell localization is associated with increased sensory innervation, and sensory hyperinnervation can aid in distinguishing overactive bladder from bladder pain syndrome histologically [6].

P.M. Hanno et al. (eds.), *Bladder Pain Syndrome – An Evolution*,
https://doi.org/10.1007/978-3-319-61449-6_24

24.3 Where Do We Go from Here?

A review of the literature does not reveal any subsequent research connecting BPS to ECP in the past 3 decades. While its potential as a fecal biomarker to reflect the colorectal inflammation seen both macroscopically and on a cellular level in ulcerative colitis has suggested the potential of ECP to be a potential detector of subclinical inflammation in that disorder [7], similar utility in BPS remains to be determined. For now, urinary eosinophilic cationic protein appears to be an interesting dead-end in the continuing search for a biomarker.

References

1. Koh GC, Shek LP, Goh DY, Van Bever H, Koh DS. Eosinophil cationic protein: is it useful in asthma? A systematic review. Respir Med. 2007;101(4):696–705.
2. Goseva Z, Janeva EJ, Gjorcev A, Arsovski Z, Pejkovska S. Role and significance of markers of inflammation in the asthmatic disease. Open Access Maced J Med Sci. 2015;3(4):630–4.
3. Shoji M, Shoji J, Inada N. Clinical severity and tear biomarkers, eosinophil cationic protein and CCL23, in chronic allergic conjunctival diseases. Semin Ophthalmol. 2016;8:1–6.
4. Topic RZ, Dodig S. Eosinophil catonic protein—current concepts and controversies. Biochem Med (Zagreb). 2011;21:111–21.
5. Gamper M, Regauer S, Welter J, Eberhard J, Viereck V. Are mast cells still good biomarkers for bladder pain syndrome/interstitial cystitis? J Urol. 2015;193(6):1994–2000.
6. Regauer S, Gamper M, Fehr MK, Viereck V. Sensory hyperinnervation distinguishes bladder pain syndrome/interstitial cystitis from overactive bladder syndrome. J Urol. 2016;197:159–66.
7. Peterson CGB, Lampinen M, Hansson T, Lidén M, Hällgren R, Carlson M. Evaluation of biomarkers for ulcerative colitis comparing two sampling methods: fecal markers reflect colorectal inflammation both macroscopically and on a cellular level. Scand J Clin Lab Invest. 2016;76(5):393–401.

The Use of Pentosan Polysulfate in the Management of Interstitial Cystitis

25

Robert M. Moldwin

"Interstitial Cystitis" was published in 1988 by Springer Verlag, and was one of the earliest publications detailing the potential role of pentosan polysulfate for the treatment of interstitial cystitis [1]. In an earlier pilot study, Parsons et al., described that this sulfated polysaccharide could improve symptoms in 90% of interstitial cystitis patients [2]. The textbook chapter that followed described the theoretical basis of pentosan polysulfate's (PPS) action along with data developed from a placebo controlled double-blinded cross over study. Results were not quite as spectacular, but nevertheless promising with 47% of PPS treated patients reporting overall symptom improvement compared to 23% of those receiving placebo. Over the past 35 years, our use of PPS in IC therapy has evolved based upon newer literature and the clinical experience of dedicated practitioners.

25.1 What's Happened to PPS Since the Publication of "Interstitial Cystitis"

Pentosan polysulfate, brand name Elmiron®, was approved in the United States for the "relief of bladder pain or discomfort associated with interstitial cystitis" in 1996 under the FDA's orphan products program (at that time, IC was considered to be a rare disorder). Package labeling details [3] describe two early studies that led to approval. The first study detailed a randomized placebo controlled trial accruing IC patients meeting strict criteria as defined by the National Institutes of Diabetes and Digestive and Kidney Diseases (NIDDK) [4] in which 151 patients were evaluated. 28/74 (38%) of patients who received PPS, 100 mg TID, and 13/74 (18%) of patients who received placebo showed greater than 50% improvement in bladder pain ($p = 0.005$).

The second study was a retrospective open label analysis of 2499 patients who received PPS, 300 mg per day. These patients, 60% of whom had severe or unbearable symptoms, were asked to rate overall change in pain in comparison to baseline at 3-month intervals. At 3 months, 1307 (52%) of the patients had dropped out or were ineligible for analysis. At the one-year mark, only 598 (24%) patients were still receiving the medication. Improvement in pain was identified by 722/2499 (29%) of the patients at 3 months. Of the 892 patients who continued taking PPS for 6 months, an additional 116/2499 (5%) of patients reported less pain. Few additional favorable responses were noted after 6 months.

Subsequent studies analyzing the role of PPS for the treatment of IC symptoms have had disparate outcomes (Table 25.1) [5–17], likely owing to differences in study design and patient population

R.M. Moldwin
Hofstra Northwell School of Medicine, Pelvic Pain Treatment Center, The Arthur Smith Institute for Urology, 450 Lakeville Road, Suite M41, Lake Success, NY 11042, USA
e-mail: rmoldwin@gmail.com

P.M. Hanno et al. (eds.), *Bladder Pain Syndrome – An Evolution*,
https://doi.org/10.1007/978-3-319-61449-6_25

Table 25.1 Studies Examining the Efficacy of PPS

Authors	Year	Study type	N	Notable findings
Parsons [2]	1983	Pilot, open label	24	22 of 24 patients (91.6%) reported symptom improvement
Parsons [1]	1984	RCT crossover		47% of patients in treatment arm improved; 23% favorable response in placebo group
Parsons and Mulholland [5]	1987	RCT cross over	62	Increased voided volumes; subjective improvements in urge, frequency, pain, nocturia
				Termination of drug resulted in symptom return within 3 to 12 weeks in 80%
Holm-Bentzen et al. [6]	1987	RCT	115	No clinically significant differences in symptoms, urodynamic parameters, cystoscopic appearance and mast cell counts
Fritjofsson et al. [7]	1987	Open label	87	Improvement in urinary frequency and voided volumes in non HL patients. These improvements were not seen in those with HL
				Pain improved in both groups and this effect was stable at the 3-month follow up
Mulholland et al. [8]	1990	RCT	110	Overall improvement of greater than 25% was reported by 28% of the PPS-treated patients and by 13% of those treated with placebo. (p = 0.03)
Parsons et al. [9]	1993	RCT	148	32% of those receiving PPS showed significant improvement compared to 16% of those on placebo (p = 0.01)
				Patients on PPS experienced a significant decrease in pain and urgency (p = 0.04 and 0.01) compared to placebo
				More subjects on PPS showed an average increase of more than 20 ml in voided volume than did placebo patients (p = 0.02)
Hanno [1]	1997	Prospective, long term, open label compassionate use	2809	46% of patients dropped out within first 3 months
				42–62% of patients receiving PPS had moderate or better symptom improvement
Jepsen et al. [11]	1998	Retrospective, long term compassionate use	97	11.3% of patient continued PPS for more than 18 mo.
				Correlation of increased PPS duration of treatment to less constant pain
Sant et al. [12]	2003	RCT	60	A non-significant trend in improved global response assessment was seen in PPS group (34%) versus placebo (18%); p = 0.064
		2x2 factorial study of PPS and hydroxyzine		
Nickel et al. [13]	2005	Randomized, double blinded, dose ranging study	380	230 patient completed study
				Mean ICSI scores and PORIS improved for 300, 600, and 900 mg dosages; improvements were not dose dependent
				Symptom response appeared to improve with longer courses of therapy
Nickel et al. [14]	2008	Retrospective	128	Patients receiving therapy soon after diagnosis may do better clinically
Davis et al. [15]	2008	RCT	41	Oral PPS demonstrated 24% reduction in symptom scores as compared to combined oral PPS and intravesical PPS (46% reduction) at 12 weeks
Al-Zahrani et al. [16]	2011	Retrospective/ long-term	271	34.3% drop out
				Better results in those with significant glomerulations
				Trend toward better response in >12 mo group

Table 25.1 (continued)

Authors	Year	Study type	N	Notable findings
Nickel et al. [17]	2015	RCT	368	44% dropout
				No difference between placebo, PPS 100 mg, PPS 300 mg dosing for primary endpoint at 24 weeks
				No difference in symptom improvement between PPS naïve and non naïve patients
				Subgroup analysis of IC/BPS patients meeting NIDDK criteria demonstrated highest response in placebo group (50%)

(Table 25.2). As seen in earlier studies, patient drop out tended to be high. An excellent review article by Propert et al. [18], which remains timely despite its 2002 publication, detailed the many dilemmas encountered in the creation of a clinical trial for any new interstitial cystitis therapy.

25.2 More Stumbling Blocks for PPS Studies

Data from recent studies of the Multidisciplinary Approaches to the Study of Chronic Urologic Pelvic Pain (MAPP) Network, an NIH supported, multi-institutional, interdisciplinary collaborative group, may have bearing upon how we interpret past research and design future studies. One MAPP investigation set off concern for significant symptom variability and a rapid regression to the mean for patients who begin clinical protocols [19]. Failure to account for these phenomena in uncontrolled studies may falsely increase the number of responders and decrease the numbers of patients who don't respond or worsen. The investigators ultimately suggested a run in period of 4 weeks or more to account for this effect.

The MAPP network also examined efficacy of the "instruments" that we have used to detect clinical changes [20]. Almost all assessments in the past have relied upon patient questionnaires that combined multiple domains, i.e., pain, urinary urgency, quality of life etc., into one total score. These investigators challenged that concept and found pain and urinary symptoms to function as independent variables when it comes to factors such as depression. They placed caution on the use of combined scores for future clinical studies.

Table 25.2 Variations between studies examining effect of PPS

• Study type and analysis
Retrospective
Open label, prospective
Open label, retrospective
Randomized, double-blind, placebo controlled
Dose ranging (varied double blinded doses, no placebo)
• Sample size
• Length of study
• Population studied
Patients meeting NIDDK criteria and those without meeting those criteria
Patients with and without Hunner lesions
PPS naïve and those that had previously used the medication
Use of concomitant therapies
• Measures of success
O'Leary Sant symptom index (ICSI)
O'Leary Sant problem index (ICPI)
University of Wisconsin interstitial cystitis scale
Global response assessment (GRA)
Patient overall rating of improvement of symptoms (PORIS)
Pain, urgency, frequency score (PUF)
Likert pain scale
Urodynamic parameters
Voiding diary (urinary frequency and voided volumes)
Health related quality of life (QoL) measures
• Other factors having an impact upon data interpretation
Intent to treat (treating patient drop outs as failures)
Selection bias (tertiary care centers versus community practice)
Regression to mean
Degree of improvement that constitutes success

Perhaps one of the most challenging aspects of developing trials for PPS (or for that matter, any therapy for IC/BPS) is the condition's phenotypic heterogeneity. While it's clear that some patients only have bladder pain, the majority do not [21]. Often patients are plagued with conditions such as irritable bowel syndrome, vulvodynia, pelvic floor myalgia, amongst many others; any of which may account for some portion of their pelvic pain … if not the majority of their pain. Those identified with non-urological causes of pelvic pain trended towards poorer quality of life, depression, and sleep disturbances [22]. Krieger and the MAPP network determined that individuals with chronic urological pain syndromes (IC/BPS and chronic prostatitis/chronic pelvic pain syndrome) had more severe urological symptoms and more frequent depression and anxiety [23]. And then there is the patient with Hunner lesions. These patients have many clinical characteristics, most notably, gross inflammatory disease of the bladder wall, that perhaps puts them in a therapeutically distinct group, one that often favors more aggressive management [5].

With all of the above variables in play, it's often difficult to make definitive statements about PPS effectiveness. An example of these difficulties can be appreciated in a recent phase 4, randomized, double–blind placebo controlled trial evaluating the efficacy of PPS for IC/BPS therapy [17]. The study found *no statistically significant difference for the primary endpoint, defined as a 30% or greater reduction from the baseline ICSI total score between 2 different doses of PPS (100 mg QD and 100 mg TID) and a placebo group*. In this well-constructed study that included intent to treat analysis, the investigators used a less rigorous definition of IC/BPS for enrollment (although sub stratification for patients meeting NIDDK criteria was also performed). They did not exclude patients with co-morbid conditions such as irritable bowel syndrome, pelvic floor dysfunction, or depression. Likewise, patients were not excluded if they had already used PPS in their clinical care. Hence, these and other factors (such as drop out for reasons other than non response to therapy and adverse events) may have inadvertently selected patients who were less likely to be responders.

The optimal dosing of PPS was evaluated in a different phase 4, double-blind, double-dummy, parallel-group multicenter 32-week trial with no placebo control. The response to treatment for doses of 300, 600, and 900 mg per day was found to be clinically significant and improved over time. On the other hand, the response to therapy was not dose dependent [13].

25.3 So What Have These Studies Along with 21 Years of Clinical Use Taught Us …?

1. PPS appears to be effective for many patients with IC/BPS but the specific phenotype of the individual most likely to respond remains unknown.
2. Clinical experience and some studies suggest a poorer response in those patients with more severe disease, i.e., Hunner lesions, and in those whose symptoms have been present for many years.
3. PPS may take 3 months (and on relatively rare occasions up to 6 months) to see efficacy. This factor may be one of the most problematic in terms of patient drop out in research studies and in clinical practice.
4. PPS dosing remains 100 mg TID, however, optimal dosing has not been determined.
5. PPS may not have significant effect on symptoms if other forms of pelvic pain, i.e., pelvic floor myalgia, endometriosis, are present and significant.
6. No published literature exists regarding the recurrence of symptoms upon discontinuance of PPS.

25.4 In Conclusion …

Trials to evaluate the efficacy of PPS are terribly difficult to construct owing to multiple factors such as the phenotypic heterogeneity of the patient population, high patient drop out, definitions of success and failure, amongst others. Most literature still favors a therapeutic role for PPS; however, several recent well-constructed studies suggest that the medication's effect may not be as robust as initially hoped. Clinical experience suggests best results are achieved in conjunction with other conservative treatment strategies.

References

1. Parsons CL. Interstitial cystitis. Use of pentosan polysulfate in the management of interstitial cystitis. In: Hanno PM, Staskin DR, Krane RJ, Wein AJ, editors. Interstitial cystitis (chapter 17). London: Springer; 1988. p. 163–8.
2. Parsons CL, Schmidt JD, Pollen JJ. Successful treatment of interstitial cystitis with sodium pentosanpolysulfate. J Urol. 1983;130:51–3.
3. http://www.accessdata.fda.gov/drugsatfda_docs/label/2008/020193s009lbl.pdf
4. Gillenwater JY, Wein AJ. Summary of the National Institute of arthritis, diabetes, digestive and kidney diseases workshop on interstitial cystitis, National Institutes of Health, Bethesda, Maryland, August 28-29, 1987. J Urol. 1988;140:203–6.
5. Parsons CL, Mulholland SG. Successful therapy of interstitial cystitis with pentosanpolysulfate. J Urol. 1987;138:513–6.
6. Holm-Bentzen M, Jacobsen F, Nerstrøm B, et al. A prospective double-blind clinically controlled multicenter trial of sodium pentosanpolysulfate in the treatment of interstitial cystitis and related painful bladder disease. J Urol. 1987;138:503–7.
7. Fritjofsson A, Fall M, Juhlin R, et al. Treatment of ulcer and nonulcer interstitial cystitis with sodium pentosanpolysulfate: a multicenter trial. J Urol. 1987;138:508–12.
8. Mulholland SG, Hanno P, Parsons CL, et al. Pentosan polysulfate sodium for therapy of interstitial cystitis. A double-blind placebo-controlled clinical study. Urology. 1990;35:552–8.
9. Parsons CL, Benson G, Childs SJ, et al. A quantitatively controlled method to study prospectively interstitial cystitis and demonstrate the efficacy of pentosanpolysulfate. J Urol. 1993;150:845–8.
10. Hanno PM. Analysis of long-term Elmiron therapy for interstitial cystitis. Urology. 1997;49:93–9.
11. Jepsen JV, Sall M, Rhodes PR, et al. Long-term experience with pentosanpolysulfate in interstitial cystitis. Urology. 1998;51:381–7.
12. Sant GR, Propert KJ, Hanno PM, et al. A pilot clinical trial of oral pentosan polysulfate and oral hydroxyzine in patients with interstitial cystitis. J Urol. 2003;170:810–5.
13. Nickel JC, Barkin J, Forrest J, et al. Randomized, double-blind, dose-ranging study of pentosan polysulfate sodium for interstitial cystitis. Urology. 2005;65:654–8.
14. Nickel JC, Kaufman DM, Zhang HF, et al. Time to initiation of pentosan polysulfate sodium treatment after interstitial cystitis diagnosis: effect on symptom improvement. Urology. 2008;71:57–61.
15. Davis EL, Khoudary el SR, Talbott EO, et al. Safety and efficacy of the use of intravesical and oral pentosan polysulfate sodium for interstitial cystitis: a randomized double-blind clinical trial. J Urol. 2008;179:177–85.
16. Al-Zahrani AA, Gajewski JB. Long-term efficacy and tolerability of pentosan polysulphate sodium in the treatment of bladder pain syndrome. Can Urol Assoc J. 2011;5:113–8.
17. Nickel JC, Herschorn S, Whitmore KE, et al. Pentosan polysulfate sodium for treatment of interstitial cystitis/bladder pain syndrome: insights from a randomized, double-blind, placebo controlled study. J Urol. 2015;193:857–62.
18. Propert KJ, Payne C, Kusek JW, Nyberg LM. Pitfalls in the design of clinical trials for interstitial cystitis. Urology. 2002;60:742–8.
19. Stephens-Shields AJ, Clemens JQ, Jemielita T, et al. Symptom variability and early symptom regression in the MAPP study: a prospective study of urological chronic pelvic pain syndrome. J Urol. 2016;196:1450–5.
20. Griffith JW, Stephens-Shields AJ, Hou X, et al. Pain and urinary symptoms should not be combined into a single score: psychometric findings from the MAPP research network. J Urol. 2016;195:949–54.
21. Nickel JC, Tripp DA, Pontari M, et al. Interstitial cystitis/painful bladder syndrome and associated medical conditions with an emphasis on irritable bowel syndrome, fibromyalgia and chronic fatigue syndrome. J Urol. 2010;184:1358–63.
22. Nickel JC, Tripp DA, International Interstitial Cystitis Study Group. Clinical and psychological parameters associated with pain pattern phenotypes in women with interstitial cystitis/bladder pain syndrome. J Urol. 2015;193:138–44.
23. Krieger JN, Stephens AJ, Clemens JQ, et al. Relationship between chronic nonurological associated somatic syndromes and symptom severity in urological chronic pelvic pain syndromes: baseline evaluation of the MAPP study. J Urol. 2015;193:1254–62.

Etiology of Interstitial Cystitis and the Role of Pentosanpolysulfate in IC Therapy

26

C. Lowell Parsons

26.1 Introduction

For over 40 years I have studied the bladder epithelium and interstitial cystitis (IC). I have seen over 9000 patients and conducted extensive basic laboratory and clinical research on IC that has substantially changed my concepts of the disease. My understanding now is that there is one primary disease process that generates bladder symptoms of urgency, frequency, pain and incontinence (in any combination) in women of all ages and men less than 55 (before the age of bladder outlet obstruction). This pathologic process is a dysfunctional, "leaky" bladder epithelium that allows urinary potassium to diffuse into the bladder interstitium and directly depolarize, nerves, muscles, cause bladder symptoms and injure tissue. The rare but not separate severe form of this process is the patient historically diagnosed with IC [1].

Six major discoveries lead to my new concepts of IC.

1. Bladder surface mucus, sometimes called the GAG layer, protects the transitional epithelium from bacterial, protein and calcium adherence providing a universal protective anti-adherence barrier [2, 3].
2. The GAG layer controls the permeability of the epithelium to small molecules in rodents and in normal human volunteers [4, 5].
3. IC patients have a leaky epithelium compared to normal human subjects to both urea and potassium [6, 7].
4. The GAG layer injured chemically in both rodents and humans results in a leaky epithelium and this injury is reversed by both heparin and pentosanpolysulfate (PPS, Elmiron) [2, 4, 5, 7–10]. This discovery led to the use of PPS to treat IC and became the first and to date only FDA approved oral medical therapy for IC [5, 8–13].
5. The discovery of the role potassium plays in the generation of bladder symptoms. If the GAG layer is defective, "leaky", urine potassium will diffuse into the bladder wall,

Comment: In the original Chapter that I wrote for this book on Pentosanpolysulfate (PPS) therapy I began with a comment that not much was known about IC etiology and go on to describe the rationale for the use of PPS in IC and its success rates. Compared to 28 years ago my concepts about interstitial cystitis have changed dramatically on the basis of new and solid scientific evidence. Substantial progress was made in the understanding of the etiology of IC, the mechanism of action for PPS in the disease as well as the potential new uses of PPS in bladder symptoms in general. There were so many changes and so much new information that I needed to rewrite the chapter (and this is a good thing) so that I could adequately explain all of these changes. The significant progress over the past three decades is self evident when the chapters are compared. I found redoing this chapter to be quiet fascinating.
C. Lowell Parsons

C. Lowell Parsons
Emeritus Professor of Surgery/Urology, School of Medicine, University of California San Diego, La Jolla, CA, USA
e-mail: cparsons@ucsd.edu

P.M. Hanno et al. (eds.), *Bladder Pain Syndrome – An Evolution*,
https://doi.org/10.1007/978-3-319-61449-6_26

depolarize muscles, nerves and cause symptoms and tissue injury. A potassium sensitivity test (PST)was developed to identify the presence of a leaky epithelium, normal subjects are not sensitive to intravesical potassium but those with a leaky bladder epithelium are [14]. Symptomatic patient populations were tested and found to have lower urinary dysfunctional epithelium (LUDE) including IC, radiation cystitis, urethral syndrome, overactive bladder, prostatitis, gynecologic chronic pelvic pain patients, vulvodynia and endometriosis and all were equally potassium sensitive [1, 7, 14–22]. Table 26.1 contains the summation of the data from over 40 studies in the world literature. These data are creating an entirely new paradigm for both urology and gynecology patients concerning bladder symptoms and chronic pelvic pain. Bottom line is all of these patients have LUDE and see specialists urologists or gynecologists based on the symptoms bothering them the most and receive a myriad of traditional diagnoses (or misdiagnoses if you will) but in reality all have only one basic disease process. Bottom line the PST is the best and most widely substantiated diagnostic test for IC/epithelial dysfunction (LUDE) with a 81% sensitivity and 99% specificity.

6. The recent identification of toxic urinary cationic metabolites that bind to and injure the GAG layer and initiate the epithelial dysfunction cascade. Most of them are nucleic acid metabolites and are very toxic to cultured urothelial cells. These urine cations are 2.5 times higher in the urine of IC patients compared to control subjects and are neutralized by Tamm Horsfall Protein (THP) PPS and heparin [21, 23]. We believe these cations are the root cause of IC.

Table 26.1 KCl test results in symptomatic patient groups

Group	N	% Positive	P value[a]
IC [1, 7, 14–17, 24]	3786	81%	<0.0001
Normal subjects [7, 14–17]	228	1.3%	
OAB [25]	116	71%	<0.0001
Prostatitis [18, 20, 22]	72	81%	<0.0001
Gyn chronic pelvic pain [16, 17, 19]	378	82%	<0.0001
Vulvodynia [19]	122	84%	<0.0001
Urethral syndrome [15]	116	55%	<0.0001
Radiation cystitis [14]	5	100%	<0.01

These data are summarized from over 40 papers in the world literature and the direct references are cited for some [1, 7, 14–22] and the rest are cited in a review article that is also referenced [19]

[a]All Groups compared to the control group

26.2 Pentosanpolysulfate

As mentioned, chemical injury of the normal bladder surface mucus will cause an injury to the barrier effect of the epithelium [2–5, 7–10]. It was also discovered that this injury in both rodents and humans can be reversed with an intravesical treatment of the bladder surface with either heparin of pentosanpolysulfate (PPS) [2, 4, 5, 7–10, 26]. As a direct result of these observations it was hypothesized that heparinoids might beneficially impact on diseases where the mucosa was dysfunctional such as interstitial cystitis. PPS has an oral form that is about 2.5% bio-available. It was then tried in several opened labeled and a double blind study [13] to determine if it had efficacy in IC and the drug was successful at relieving symptoms after several months of therapy [27, 28]. Bear in mind that in the early 1980s when these initial studies were done IC for the most part was only recognized in its severe form where symptoms were chronic and unrelenting. It was 20 plus years later that IC was indeed discovered to have a beginning where symptoms are mild and intermittent [29]. And In this early phase is far more common than the rare severe but classical form of IC. So the initial experience with IC was on the severe patients and the positive results that were obtained were quite promising. These studies led to key pivotal clinical trials. The company conducting the trials met with the United States Food and Drug Administration (FDA) and developed a protocol that was acceptable to the FDA. Basically the two trials were randomized, prospective, multicentered placebo controlled trials. The entry criteria were strictly defined and utilized the NIDDK criteria which were developed shortly before these clinical trials began. These two studies used the the Global Assessment Response of symptoms (known as the GAR) as the primary outcome measure which was first reported by Parsons [13]. The GAR was statistically validated as an outcome measure for IC clinical trials in the larger of these two studies [12] and is now widely used for this purpose. Patients entered were defined as having severe disease for at least 1 year with moderate or worse symptoms of pain and urgency, had a cystoscopy under anesthesia, completed a 3 day voided log (at the beginning and end of the trial) and were begun on PPS 100 mg TID for 3 months. At the end of the study the global assessment of symptoms questionnaire was filled out by each patient. It is a six point scale with patients reporting (1) worse (2) 0% improved (3) 25% improved (4) 50% improved (5) 75% improved (6) 100% improved. Better was predefined in the protocols as 50% or greater improvement and those not reaching this level were deemed no better. The percent of patients reporting better is summarized in Table 26.2 for each study. These studies were the basis for approval of PPS to treat IC by the Food and Drug Administration in the United States in 1996.

26.3 Dose of Pentosanpolysulfate for Therapy

PPS should be the basis for any single or multimodal therapy for IC since it treats the root cause of IC the epithelial dysfunction [30]. Severe patients usually require the multiple therapy approach to address both the epithelial problem and their symptoms. The approved dosage of PPS is 300 mg per day. A subsequent study showed that longer durations of therapy up to 8 months resulted in a higher success rate of improvements in patients up to 70% [31]. Currently, I routinely start female patients on 200 mg of PPS BID and if not better in 4 months increase the dose to 300 mg BID. For severe patients if not better at 6–8 months I will increase it to 300 mg TID. Males I routinely start on 300 mg BID. I never stop the PPS until the patients lose all or most of the symptoms but frequently add other therapies to control their symptoms. In general PPS (or other heparinoids) are the only drugs the reverse the course of the disease and reduce the epithelial leak of potassium allowing the bladder to heal [30]. It should always be the primary foundation of therapy. It is important to have patience and continue therapy and encourage people (especially patients with many years of severe symptoms) to stay on treatment indefinitely even years before success may be obtained. Explaining to the patient that PPS can reverse the course of the disease is helpful so that they realize that staying on the medication is critical along with other treatment modalities that may be added to their therapeutic regimen. PPS has been on the Unites States market for over 20 years. This long experience with the drug has shown that it is very benign and well tolerated and has been used in well over 100,000 people with an excellent safety profile in both the low and high doses of medication reported herein.

I have reported successful use of PPS in 42 children and the dose by weight that I have employed is presented in Table 26.3 [32]. In General children responded quicker and better to therapy which is probably not surprising since

Table 26.2 Summary of two pivotal PPS trials

	N	Placebo GAR*	Drug GAR*	P value[a, b]
Mulholland 1990 [11]				
Overall improved	110	13%%	28%	0.04
Pain improved		14%	27%	0.08
Pressure to urinate improved		11%	22%	0.08
Parsons 1993 [12]				
Overall improved	148	15%	36%	0.002
Pain improved		18%	38%	0.005
Pressure to urinate improved		18%	30%	0.04

[a]GAR is the global assessment response In both studies drug did significantly better that placebo. These studies were the basis for FDA approval in the USA in 1996 of PPS for treating IC

[b]Compares active drug to placebo

Table 26.3 Dose of PPS for use in children by weight

Weight (lbs)	Dose
25–45	50 mg BID[a]
45–70	100 mg BID
70	200 mg BID

[a]If child cannot take a pill empty capsule into 1 ounce of water and have the child drink it. PPS is acid stable and not affected by the stomach

they have had disease for a shorter time and tend to heal faster than do adults.

26.4 Mechanism of Pentosanpolysulfate Action

Since intravesical PPS will restore an experimentally injured GAG layer in either normal rodents or adult humans the hypothesis for its mechanism of action in IC patients was that in restores the GAG layer by coating the bladder surface [7, 10, 30]. But more recently our discoveries of cations in urine that injure the GAG layer has led to a new and/or additional hypothesis [21, 23].

I believe that "sometimes the obvious is the reality" and in the case of IC that urine is the cause of the disease, not the nerves, spinal cord, pelvic floor or other systemic remote issues. If there were no urine in the bladder then no disease would exist. IC has a beginning usually early in the life of most patients (by ages 18–25) [29] with mild and intermittent symptoms and in the unfortunate individuals progresses over decades to a more chronic and debilitating condition. It is the older patients with years of more severe disease that develop associated problems secondary to the chronic disease process such as e.g. pelvic floor dysfunction. So what starts the disease process? What causes the GAG layer to become dysfunctional?

The urinary bladder has a hostile environment to deal with namely urine and the toxic byproducts of metabolism it contains. Fortunately the marvelous impermeable GAG layer confines them to the bladder lumen for the most part rendering them harmless. But this is not always the case. IC patients have a dysfunctional GAG layer and as a consequence the highly concentrated urinary potassium levels are allowed to diffuse into the bladder wall and depolarize muscles, nerves and ultimately destroy tissue [1]. A key question is what causes the GAG layer to become abnormal? Our hypothesis has been that urinary cationic metabolites containing amino groups will bind to and impair the function of this layer similar to what protamine does in normal rodents and humans where it causes a leaky epithelium [4–7]. Based on this hypothesis, all urinary cationic molecules were isolated from urine of normal human subjects using ion-exchange cartridges in attempt to determine if it contained these postulated toxins. The positively charged compounds were isolated and identified by using a combination of high performance liquid chromatography (HPLC) and mass spectroscopy (MS) [21]. Once these molecules were identified they were purchase commercially and used in cell cultures of bladder epithelial cells to determine if they would injure and kill the cells. For a positive control protamine (very cytotoxic to the cultured cells) was used and compared on a weight basis to the isolated urinary cations for cytotoxicity. Four of these cations were found to be very toxic and surprisingly turned out to be metabolites of DNA and they are significantly elevated in the urine of IC patients [21]. The entire cation content was extracted from the urine of both normal subjects and IC patients. The toxic cations were over two fold increased in the urine of the IC patients [21, 23].When the fractions of cations from both groups were compared in our cytotoxicity assay, all of the patient fractions were more toxic than all of the normal subjects and hence by definition a good diagnostic test [21]. Another study on the cation content in urine was conducted that compared patients with active symptoms to patients significantly improved on PPS therapy and both groups had the same elevated levels compared to control subjects [23]. These data are important because it seems that these cations are not a result of the IC disease process since they do not go down at all when patients are significantly improved. The discovery of these toxic cationic metabolites is a major and very important piece of the IC puzzle. We believe that these toxic

DNA metabolites injure the bladder GAG layer by binding to it and begin the whole IC cascade. The cytotoxicity of the whole cation fractions, as well as, the individual toxic compounds from patients and control subjects was exposed to both Tamm Horsfall Protein and PPS and each compound completely neutralized the toxic effect of these cations. The ability of PPS to sequester these toxic cations is probably the mechanism for the activity of PPS in urine and explains why it is successful in treating IC patients. Some of my patients with severe IC symptoms have over four times the cation levels of normal people and explains why we have found these patients do better if prescribed much higher doses of PPS.

The role that toxic urinary cations may play in the initiation of bladder symptoms and IC opens the door for the development of new drugs that target these metabolites for sequestration. Determining the cation levels in patients, particularly severe ones, will help guide therapy by increasing the presence in urine a level of medication necessary to effectively neutralize these toxins. Since PPS is very capable of performing this task what is needed is a form of PPS that has better gastrointestinal absorption to deliver higher levels of this drug to the urine that will likely result in a much higher rate of improvement in patients. It is interesting that PPS was the first and currently only approved oral drug for IC in the United States and the new understanding of its mechanism of action shows that the original hypothesis to use it in IC was essentially correct. And that a new drug does not necessarily need to be developed to do the same thing what needs to be accomplished is delivering more PPS to the urinary tract.

The Combination of epithelial dysfunction or LUDE disease and potassium problems occur in many patients with bladder symptoms (e.g. OAB, prostatitis) and gynecologic chronic pelvic pain. PPS therapy may be very useful in these patient populations no matter what their classical diagnosis is. Interestingly, PPS was introduced in IC patients at a time when the disease was considered rare but it may be the therapeutic of choice for tens of millions of patients with bladder and pelvic pain symptoms based primarily on new understandings of the etiology of bladder symptoms and its mechanisms of action in the urinary tract.

References

1. Parsons CL. The role of a leaky epithelium and potassium in the generation of bladder symptoms in interstitial cystitis/overactive bladder, urethral syndrome, prostatitis and gynaecological chronic pelvic pain. BJU Int. 2011;107:370–5.
2. Parsons CL, Stauffer C, Schmidt JD. Bladder-surface glycosaminoglycans: an efficient mechanism of environmental adaptation. Science. 1980;208(4444):605–7.
3. Parsons CL, Greenspan C, Mulholland SG. The primary antibacterial defense mechanism of the bladder. Investig Urol. 1975;13(1):72–8.
4. Parsons CL, et al. Bladder surface glycosaminoglycans: an epithelial permeability barrier. J Urol. 1990;143(1):139–42.
5. Lilly JD, Parsons CL. Bladder surface glycosaminoglycans is a human epithelial permeability barrier. Surg Gynecol Obstet. 1990;171(6):493–6.
6. Parsons CL, Lilly JD, Stein P. Epithelial dysfunction in nonbacterial cystitis (interstitial cystitis). J Urol. 1991;145(4):732–5.
7. Parsons CL, et al. The role of urinary potassium in the pathogenesis and diagnosis of interstitial cystitis. J Urol. 1998;159(6):1862–6.
8. Parsons CL, Stauffer CW, Schmidt JD. Reversible inactivation of bladder surface glycosaminoglycan antibacterial activity by protamine sulfate. Infect Immun. 1988;56(5):1341–3.
9. Parsons CL, Mulholland SG, Anwar H. Antibacterial activity of bladder surface mucin duplicated by exogenous glycosaminoglycan (heparin). Infect Immun. 1979;24(2):552–7.
10. Parsons CL, Pollen JJ, Anwar H, Stauffer C, Schmidt JD. Antibacterial activity of bladder surface mucin duplicated in the rabbit bladder by exogenous glycosaminoglycan (sodium pentosanpolysulfate). Infect Immun. 1980;27(3):876–81.
11. Mulholland SG, Hanno P, Parsons CL, Sant GR, Staskin DR. Pentosanpolysulfate sodium for therapy of interstitial cystitis. A double-blind placebo-controlled clinical study. Urology. 1990;35(6):552–8.
12. Parsons CL, Benson G, Childs SJ, Hanno P, Sant GR, Webster GJ. A quantitatively controlled method to study prospectively interstitial cystitis and demonstrate the efficacy of pentosanpolysulfate. Urology. 1993;150(3):845–8.
13. Parsons CL, Mulholland SG. Successful therapy of interstitial cystitis with pentosanpolysulfate. J Urol. 1987;138:513–16.
14. Parsons CL, et al. Abnormal sensitivity to intravesical potassium in interstitial cystitis and radiation cystitis. Neurourol Urodyn. 1994;13(5):515–20.
15. Parsons CL, Zupkas P, Parsons JK. Intravesical potassium sensitivity in patients with interstitial cystitis

and urethral syndrome. Urology. 2001;57(3):428–32. discussion 432-3.
16. Parsons CL, et al. The prevalence of interstitial cystitis in gynecologic patients with pelvic pain, as detected by intravesical potassium sensitivity. Am J Obstet Gynecol. 2002;187(5):1395–400.
17. Parsons CL, et al. Increased prevalence of interstitial cystitis: previously unrecognized urologic and gynecologic cases identified using a new symptom questionnaire and intravesical potassium sensitivity. Urology. 2002;60(4):573–8.
18. Parsons CL, Albo M. Intravesical potassium sensitivity in patients with prostatitis. J Urol. 2002;168(3):1054–7.
19. Kahn BS, Tatro C, Parsons CL, Willems JJ. Prevalence of interstitial cystitis in vulvodynia patients detected by bladder potassium sensitivity. J Sex Med. 2010; 7(2 Pt 2):996–1002.
20. Parsons CL, et al. Quantifying symptoms in men with interstitial cystitis/prostatitis, and its correlation with potassium-sensitivity testing. BJU Int. 2005;95(1):86–90.
21. Parsons CL, Shaw T, Berecz Z, Su Y, Zupkas P, Argade S. Role of urinary cations in the aetiology of bladder symptoms and interstitial cystitis. BJU Int. 2014;114(2):286–93.
22. Hassan AA, Elgamal SA, Sabaa MA, Salem K. Evaluation of intravesical potassium sensitivity test and bladder biopsy in patients with chronicprostatitis/chronic pelvic pain syndrome. Int J Urol. 2007;14(8):738–42.
23. Argade S, Berecz Z, Su Y, Parsons CL. Increased toxic urinary cations in males with interstitial cystitis: a possible cause of bladder symptoms. World J Urol. 2016;34(12):1685–91.
24. Jiang YH, Jhang JF, Kuo HC. Revisiting the role of potassium sensitivity testing and cystoscopic hydrodistention for the diagnosis of interstitial cystitis. PLoS One. 2016;11(3):e0151692. doi:10.1371/journal.pone.0151692.
25. Minaglia S, Ozel B, Bizhang R, Mishell DR Jr. Increased prevalence of interstitial cystitis in women with detrusor overactivity refractory to anticholinergic therapy. Urology. 2005;66(4):702–6.
26. Hanno PM, Parsons CL, Shrom SH, Fritz R, Mulholland SG. The protective effect of heparin in experimental bladder infection. J Surg Res. 1978;25(4):324–9.
27. Parsons CL, Schmidt JD, Pollen JJ. Successful treatment of interstitial cystitis with sodium pentosanpolysulfate. J Urol. 1983;130(1):51–3.
28. Holm-Bentzen M, Jacobsen F, Nerstrøm B, Lose G, Kristensen JK, Pedersen RH, Krarup T, Feggetter J, Bates P, Barnard R, et al. A prospective double-blind clinically controlled multicenter trial of sodium pentosanpolysulfate in the treatment of interstitial cystitis and related painful bladder disease. J Urol. 1987;138(3):503–7.
29. Parsons CL. How does interstitial cystitis begin? Transl Androl Urol. 2015;4(6):605–10. doi:10.3978/j.issn.2223-4683.2015.11.02.PMID:26816860.
30. Parsons CL, Forrest J, Nickel JC, Evans R, Lloyd LK, Barkin J, Mosbaugh PG, Kaufman DM, Hernandez-Graulau JM, Atkinson L, Albrecht D, Elmiron Study Group. Effect of pentosan polysulfate therapy on intravesical potassium sensitivity. Urology. 2002;59(3):329–33.
31. Nickel JC, Barkin J, Forrest J, Mosbaugh PG, Hernandez-Graulau J, Kaufman D, Lloyd K, Evans RJ, Parsons CL, Atkinson LE, Elmiron Study Group. Randomized, double-blind, dose-ranging study of pentosan polysulfate sodium for interstitial cystitis. Urology. 2005;65(4):654–8.
32. Parsons CL. Diagnosing the bladder as the source of pelvic pain: successful treatment for adults and children. Pain Manage. 2014;4(4):293–301.

Use of Transcutaneous Electrical Nerve Stimulation in the Management of Bladder Pain Syndrome

27

Magnus Fall

Our study, presented at different stages [1–3], was of a pilot character but in this connection there were a substantial number of patients, 60 men and women in the final report, published a few years after the book on Interstitial Cystitis. There were and still remain many unsolved technical issues e.g. about the most efficacious electrical parameters to use, about optimal electrode shape and positioning, including the problem how to best overcome sensory limitations of percutaneous electrical stimulation, and also about the choice of most appropriate nerve afferents for an optimal effect; stimulation efficacy depends on the size of the responsible afferent nerve and the distance to the stimulating electrode as well as the selection of optimal electrical parameters for the desired effect [4]. We used standard TENS equipment, and cannot be sure that it was best suited for the effect we aimed to attain. It is should also be noted that there were no experimental studies as to treatment with this modality on this indication. More in-depth investigation of factors mentioned above would maybe have further improved the outcome; such studies are still feasible.

Still, in spite of possible shortcomings, the overall results were surprisingly good, and to some extent unexpected, especially so in patients with Hunner disease, ESSIC type 3C [5]. From a neurophysiologic point of view, an exceptionally interesting observation was the curative effect obtained following prolonged treatment. That included relief of symptoms, paralleled by endoscopic healing, and along with a profound reduction of MCs in bladder washings. Take for instance this *case example* [3]: A previously healthy woman was diagnosed with classic interstitial cystitis at the age of 49. There were a number of treatment attempts but the only one giving alleviation (although short-lived) was cystoscopic hydrodistension under anesthesia, performed every third month during a very long period of time. At all these frequently repeated cystoscopies the typical, circumscript Hunner lesions were seen. At the age of 66 she started chronic suprapubic, high-frequency TENS. There was continuous improvement during the following year and after one and a half year she was free of symptoms. The bladder capacity at distension during anesthesia at this stage had increased to 450 mL, compared to about 240 mL, constantly, at the very numerous distensions by way of the cystoscope before starting TENS. Three years later she was reexamined and the bladder capacity now was 800 mL; she was still free of symptoms. All lesions and signs of inflammation had disappeared; the bladder mucosa exhibited a few tiny, pale scars where lesions had been situated before. She was followed for 17 years after initiation of TENS, had no relapse and continued to use her device off and on. In this context it is

M. Fall
Department of Urology Institute of Clinical Sciences, Sahlgrenska Academy at the University of Gothenburg, SE 41345 Göteborg, Sweden
e-mail: magnus.fall@urology.gu.se

P.M. Hanno et al. (eds.), *Bladder Pain Syndrome – An Evolution*,
https://doi.org/10.1007/978-3-319-61449-6_27

worth noting that spontaneous healing of Hunner lesions had not reported. In this group of patients with Hunner lesions it is also worth noting the well documented, very long duration of stable clinical signs and symptoms before TENS was initiated; TENS was the starting point of a dramatic change. Unfortunately, though, the effect of TENS was not as convincing in non-Hunner disease, a heterogenic category where good treatment options are scarce.

Electrical stimulation is a principle but not a method. It is important to understand that there are fundamental differences in how various reflex systems are activated when you chose different applications. Effects on the bladder vs the urethra, the occurrence of the so called reeducation effect etc. can change profoundly depending on parameters like electrode positioning, electrode shape and stimulation parameters [4]. TENS is not the same as pelvic floor stimulation [6].

Although the referred studies certainly indicate a role for TENS, this treatment has not gained sufficient interest to result in further studies, neither has it achieved a role in the majority of algorithms for BPS treatment. One important reason for this is the problem of scientific evidence—no RCT: s have been performed. Another reason is that there has been lack of resources for technical development and no marketing. From a principal point of view, the remarkable observations of cure still qualify for further trials. Fortunately however, other modalities of neurostimulation involving implanted electrodes have attracted much attention with a number of successful studies presented [7–9] also including randomization [9]. Neurostimulation is a wide and vital but relatively unexplored field compared to neuropharmacology. It holds promise for the future.

Points of interest:

1. Rearrangement and restoration of the micturition reflexes by means of electrical stimulation also includes activation of links between the nervous system and the immune cell system, links that could explain the curative effect noted. Such links have been demonstrated experimentally e.g. in the gut and other organ systems. Interestingly, another way of reducing pathologically increased afferent input from the bladder by long-term lidocaine treatment has also been demonstrated to result in symptom remission as well as resolution of Hunner lesions [10].
2. "Bladder contracture" in Hunner disease (ESSIC type 3C) is often but not always caused by fibrotic bladder wall changes. Reduced volume capacity during anesthesia may sometimes reflect the functional state of a bladder never allowed to fill because of pain. When that is the case "contracture" may be more or less reversible, an observation also sometimes made after TUR or other successful treatment [1].

27.1 What Did We Get Right?

The observations of the effect of TENS are principally interesting but have attained limited penetration.

27.2 Where Did We Go Off Base?

Why has a treatment so cheap, yielding such remarkable effects and being almost without side effects attracted so little attention?

Compared to surgical techniques of electrical stimulation, TENS is maybe somewhat odd in a surgical department. Lack of marketing has a great impact. Furthermore, this kind of treatment is not as easy to accomplish as one could imagine as it requires appreciable persistence and enthusiasm from the patient as well as the therapist; the patient will certainly need encouragement when starting and carrying on with TENS. A modality of this kind should perhaps be administered by pain specialists or neurologists in cooperation with specialist nurses with more experience and training administering and following up treatments like TENS.

27.3 Where Do We Go from Here?

To be accepted, treatment methods require high scoring in level of evidence to earn high grades of recommendation. Studies on TENS are scant and there is no RCT. Since TENS can have remarkable effects, is harmless and is lacking side effects, studies on TENS are still warranted and can hopefully be repeated elsewhere to corroborate or refute our results.

References

1. Fall M. Conservative management of chronic interstitial cystitis: transcutaneous electrical nerve stimulation and transurethral resection. J Urol. 1985;133:774–8.
2. Fall M. Transcutaneous electrical nerve stimulation in interstitial cystitis. Update on clinical experience. Urology. 1987;29(4 Suppl):40–2.
3. Fall M, Lindstrom S. Transcutaneous electrical nerve stimulation in classic and nonulcer interstitial cystitis. Urol Clin North Am. 1994;21(1):131–9.
4. Fall M, Lindström S. Electrical stimulation. A physiologic approach to the treatment of urinary incontinence. Urol Clin North Am. 1991;18:393–407.
5. van de Merwe JP, Nordling J, Bouchelouche P, Bouchelouche K, Cervigni M, Daha LK, et al. Diagnostic criteria, classification, and nomenclature for painful bladder syndrome/interstitial cystitis: an ESSIC proposal. Eur Urol. 2008;53(1):60–7.
6. Fall M, Carlsson CA, Erlandson BE. Electrical stimulation in interstitial cystitis. J Urol. 1980;123:192–5.
7. van Balken MR, Vandoninck V, Gisolf KW, Vergunst H, Kiemeney LA, Debruyne FM, et al. Posterior tibial nerve stimulation as neuromodulative treatment of lower urinary tract dysfunction. J Urol. 2001;166:914–8.
8. Marinkovic S, Gillen L, Marinkovic C. Minimum 6-year outcomes for interstitial cystitis treated with sacral neuromodulation. Int Urogynecol J. 2011;22(4):407–12. Epub 2010 Sep 17.
9. Peters KM, Feber KM, Bennett RC. A prospective, single-blind, randomized crossover trial of sacral vs pudendal nerve stimulation for interstitial cystitis. BJU Int. 2007;100(4):835–9.
10. Nickel JC, Jain P, Shore N, Anderson J, Giesing D, Lee H, et al. Continuous intravesical lidocaine treatment for interstitial cystitis/bladder pain syndrome: safety and efficacy of a new drug delivery device. Sci Transl Med. 2012;18(4):143.

Use of Transcutaneous Electrical Nerve Stimulation in the Management of Bladder Pain Syndrome: 2017 Update

28

Kenneth M. Peters

28.1 What Did We Get Right?

It is very interesting to look back to 1988 and realize how little was known regarding electrical stimulation or neuromodulation in the management of voiding dysfunction and pelvic pain. The original chapter had sparse data on the use of transcutaneous electrical nerve stimulation (TENS) as a means to improve symptoms of interstitial cystitis. It was suggested that other sites of stimulation such as intravaginal or posterior tibial nerve may improve clinical outcomes. The author commented that the ideal site of stimulation was unknown and research was needed to identify the best stimulation parameters to achieve good clinical outcomes. Since that time, cutaneous stimulation is routinely used, but still with little evidence. It is often physical therapists who use TENS and inferential stimulation units as a multimodal approach to managing chronic pelvic pain. There has been broadened interest in the impact of the pelvic floor and neuromuscular dysfunction as an underlying trigger for pain associated with interstitial cystitis. Thus, neuromodulation is a reasonable modality to offer patients with interstitial cystitis symptoms.

The author was insightful in proposing inhibition of bladder afferents, modulation of bladder efferents, an impact on opioid/endorphin release and perhaps a local influence on the detrusor inflammatory cell aggregates as potential mechanisms of action of electrical stimulation. Interestingly, despite years of research on neuromodulation since the book was published in 1988, we still do not have a clear understanding as to how neuromodulation works. A significant amount of research has focused on the effect of sacral neuromodulation (SNM) on afferent sensory nerve fibers, with the dominant theory being that electrical stimulation of these somatic afferent fibers modulates voiding and continence reflex pathways in the central nervous system (CNS).

The control of sensory input to the CNS is thought to work through a gate control mechanism.

The gate control theory states that noxious stimuli perception does not entirely depend on the A-delta and C-fiber sensory nerves transmitting information to the CNS, but on the pattern of peripheral nerve activity. A-delta bladder afferent nerve fibers project to the pontine nuclei to provide inhibitory and excitatory input to reflexes controlling bladder and sphincter function. Afferent C-fibers within the bladder are normally thought to be mechano-insensitive and unresponsive and

K.M. Peters, M.D.
Beaumont Health-Royal Oak,
3535 W., 13 Mile Road, Ste. 438,
Royal Oak, MI 48073, USA
e-mail: kenneth.peters@beaumont.edu

P.M. Hanno et al. (eds.), *Bladder Pain Syndrome – An Evolution*,
https://doi.org/10.1007/978-3-319-61449-6_28

thus referred to as silent C-fibers. These normally inactive C-fibers may be sensitized by inflammation or infection, thus causing activation of involuntary micturition reflexes and detrusor overactivity. Sensory input from large myelinated pudendal nerve fibers may modulate erroneous bladder input conveyed by A-delta or C-fiber afferents at the gate control level of the spinal cord. Detrusor hyperreflexia then may be attributed to a deficiency of the inhibitory control systems involving pudendal afferent nerves. The success of electrical neuromodulation for detrusor hyperreflexia may result from the restoration of the balance between bladder inhibitory and excitatory control systems. The stimulation of urethral afferents to facilitate the micturition reflex and stimulation of the dorsal nerve of the clitoris to inhibit bladder activity have been demonstrated in animal models for SNM.

28.2 Where Were We Off Base?

Since publication of the original book on interstitial cystitis, much research has been done on neuromodulation. Sacral Neuromodulation (SNM) has the most clinical data and an implantable sacral nerve stimulator was approved in the United States in 1997 for voiding dysfunction. Since that time there have been dozens of published articles on its effectiveness in interstitial cystitis/bladder pain syndrome. Unfortunately, most of these are case series without controls. However, consistently, there have been reports of reduced urinary frequency and urgency in patients with IC/BPS and most studies demonstrate a meaningful and sustained reduction in pelvic pain.

Sacral Neuromodulation impacts a single nerve root (S3), but based on the thought that neuromodulation is dependent on afferent signals being sent to the central nervous system (CNS), pudendal neuromodulation was developed and studied. The pudendal nerve comprises S2, S3 and S4. Thus, if the pudendal nerve is activated, there is enhanced afferent signaling traveling to the CNS. A randomized trial was performed comparing sacral to pudendal stimulation in patients with IC/BPS and in a blinded fashion, each patient trialed both a sacral lead and a pudendal lead. After the staged trial, 79% of patients found pudendal neuromodulation superior to sacral. Since that time, multiple reports have shown that approximately 90% of subjects not responding to SNS will respond to PNS demonstrating this nerve target should be considered for SNM failures.

In addition, the diagnosis of IC is controversial. Classic Hunner Lesion IC is clear cut, but many patients without Hunner's Lesions have a complex phenotype suggesting the bladder may be an innocent bystander in a more complex pelvic process. In our experience, the pudendal nerve and pelvic floor muscle spasm are the culprits in many of these patients. Often there is pain in the distribution of the pudendal nerve, bladder frequency, urgency and hesitancy along with dyspareunia. Patients may experience pain the vulva/vestibule and many suffer from complex disorders such as persistent genital arousal disorder (PGAD). It is our experience that the pudendal nerve drives much of these symptoms and for those who fail to have a sustained improvement using conservative therapy such as pelvic floor physical therapy, transvaginal trigger point injections and pudendal nerve blocks; pudendal neuromodulation may be an ideal treatment for these patients.

In 1988, the original chapter on interstitial cystitis briefly mentioned the tibial nerve as a potential nerve target to treat this condition. The tibial nerve is comprised of L4, L5, S1, S2 and S3. Thus, in theory, stimulating the tibial nerve may result in more afferent signaling and have an improved clinical response. Unfortunately, it is just in the recent past that this nerve target has been scientifically studied. The only sham-controlled trial on neuromodulation for overactive bladder demonstrated that stimulating the tibial nerve, 30 min, once a week for 12 weeks is effective in reducing urinary urgency and frequency. There are just a few small case reports of percutaneous tibial nerve stimulation in the management of interstitial cystitis symptoms. Most report positive results, but more robust studies are needed to recommend this nerve target for IC/BPS. Using microimplant technology with wireless energy transmission, studies are underway to evaluate the impact of chronic tibial neuromodulation on voiding dysfunction. Chronic stimulation may enhance the effect of this nerve target and if successful, future studies can be designed to study the impact of Chronic Neuromodulation of the Tibial nerve as a treatment for IC/BPS.

28.3 Where Do We Go from Here

All organs in the body are stimulated by nerves, which send signals that affect the organ's function. Modulation of nerve signals to control or correct organ function has been recognized as a potentially powerful way to treat many diseases. The authors of the original 1988 Chapter on Electrical Stimulation for the treatment of interstitial cystitis were ahead of their time. Neuromodulation, whether transcutaneous, percutaneous or implantable is now an active area of research to manage various medical conditions. The term electroceuticals is the broad term used to describe the use of neuromodulation to manage disease. There is a coordinated effort through the NIH SPARC initiative and in partnership with industry to enhance our understanding of ideal nerve targets, develop micro-implants, create active feedback loops to improve clinical outcomes and broaden our understanding of neuromodulation in the management of various medical conditions. The future of neuromodulation for the management of interstitial cystitis/pelvic pain symptoms is exciting!

Bibliography

1. Marinkovic SP, Gillen LM, Marinkovic CM. Minimum 6-year outcomes for interstitial cystitis treated with sacral neuromodulation. Int Urogynecol J. 2011;22(4):407-412.
2. Peters KM, Feber KM, Bennett RC. A prospective single-blind, randomized crossover trial of sacral vs pudendal nerve stimulation for interstitial cystitis. BJU Int. 2007;100(4):835–9.
3. Tai C, et al. Differential role of opioid receptors in tibial nerve inhibition of nociceptive and nonnociceptive bladder reflexes in cats. Am J Physiol Renal Physiol. 2012;302(9):F1090–7.
4. Peters KM, Carrico DJ, Perez-Marrero RA, Khan AU, Wooldridge LS, Davis GL, MacDiarmid SA. Randomized trial of percutaneous tibial nerve stimulation versus sham efficacy in the treatment of overactive bladder syndrome: results from the SUmiT trial. J Urol. 2010;183(4):1438–43.
5. Kabay S, et al. Efficiency of posterior tibial nerve stimulation in category IIIB chronic prostatitis/chronic pelvic pain: a Sham-Controlled Comparative Study. Urol Int. 2009;83(1):33–8.
6. van Balken MR, et al. Percutaneous tibial nerve stimulation as neuromodulative treatment of chronic pelvic pain. Eur Urol. 2003;43(2):158–63.
7. Fitzgerald MP, Payne DK, Lukacz ES, Yang CC, Peters KM, Chai TC, et al. Randomized multicenter clinical trial of myofascial physical therapy in women with interstitial cystitis/painful bladder syndrome and pelvic floor tenderness. J Urol. 2012;187(6):2113–8.
8. Peters KM, Killinger KA, Jaeger C, Chen C. Pilot study exploring chronic pudendal neuromodulation as a treatment option for pain associated with pudendal neuralgia. Low Urin Tract Symptoms. 2015;7(3):138–42. doi:10.1111/luts.12066.
9. Liberman D, Singh R, Siegel SW. Neuromodulation for pelvic pain and sexual dysfunction. Curr Bladder Dysfunct Rep. 2016;11(2):187–93.

29 Reappraisal of Transurethral Resection in Classic Interstitial Cystitis

Magnus Fall

The idea of removing Hunner lesions to improve symptoms is not new. Guy Hunner himself found that resection of lesions was one means to obtain symptom remission, although mostly short-lived so he gave up this kind of treatment. TUR was on trial more recently [1, 2] but this kind of surgery was not accepted when we started our first series. Initially, when applying TUR our goals were twofold: to obtain sufficient tissue to permit a reliable and sufficiently detailed histopathological diagnosis, and also to establish whether careful resection of lesions actually could help patients. At this stage there was some skepticism, with questions like: if you have an ulcer and by an operation create an even bigger ulcer, how is it possible that such a measure would make any improvement? There are reasonable explanations, though [3, 4]: peripheral denervation with removal of inflamed nerve endings, reduction of aggregates of potent inflammatory mediators and elimination of epithelial mast cell recruiting factors as well as epithelial and subepithelial mast cells might cause disease remission. In this context it is worth noting that perineural localization of inflammatory cells is a very typical feature in classic interstitial cystitis [5]. At the initial stage there was also much uncertainty about what Hunner lesions really look like [6] and certainly about their prevalence. Prevalence was thought to be in the range of 5–10% of subjects with bladder pain while in our series it is around 50% [7, 8]. Recent reports indicate that the use of cystoscopy and bladder distension as a routine in BPS/IC—or lack of such routine—is decisive for the number of patients with Hunner lesion you detect or miss. In centers where the traditional way of diagnostics was not abandoned prevalence similar to ours has been reported. Fortunately, the role of cystoscopy is now increasingly appreciated worldwide [9, 10].

The electrical settings were on the lowest intensity possible, still effective for resection, and there was only pin-point coagulation of bleeding vessels with no coagulation over large surfaces, with the intention to minimize development of scar tissue that could promote bladder contracture [3]. That makes the operation technically challenging and now and then also time-consuming since, based on experience, it is important to identify all lesions and remove all involved areas including the peripheral edema zone; completeness is crucial for the result. That is a limitation of this technique since it takes a very experienced surgeon to perform mostly multiple, wide resections over the entire bladder area, typically including the dome, on thin-walled bladders. Simple coagulation of lesions is much easier but carries its own downside, since radical wide coagulation in an organ prone to contraction seems risky. It is reasonable to

M. Fall
Department of Urology, Institute of Clinical Sciences, Sahlgrenska Academy at the University of Gothenburg, SE-41345 Göteborg, Sweden
e-mail: magnus.fall@urology.gu.se

P.M. Hanno et al. (eds.), *Bladder Pain Syndrome – An Evolution*,
https://doi.org/10.1007/978-3-319-61449-6_29

believe that the result of TUR would be better and more durable, with less risk of inducing bladder contracture, although admittedly a reasoning of probability since at this stage there are no comparative studies. It is also worth noting that in a recent large series coagulation did not result in bladder volume decrease [11]. When comparing various reports duration of symptom relief seems to be longer following TUR.

The hitherto largest series [4] confirm the remarkable efficacy of this treatment, 92 of 103 patients having remission of symptoms after TUR, and long-term relief. Ablative treatment has stood the test of time and is today standard treatment with no need of justification as first line treatment of classic interstitial cystitis (ESSIC type 3C) [12].

29.1 What Did We Get Right?

The pioneering initiative by the NIH/NIDDK to establish scientific criteria for IC, presented in the book of 1990, drew attention to IC and in the following years a large number of articles were published. It was gradually realized, however, that chronic pelvic pain encompasses not only a large group of individuals but also a number of conditions lacking consensus definition criteria; very important notions. At this stage there was a conflict between the expansion of the target group and the lack of scientific clarity and transparency when grouping together a variety of conditions and syndromes with similar symptoms as their principal common feature. We began to realize that IC, for example, does not only represent one disease, but rather various subtypes or even various diseases. All treatments cannot be expected to work in all subjects. Adequate phenotyping is the key to success.

29.2 What Seminal Publications Changed Our Thinking?

Our contribution was to point out and further illustrate the multiple characteristics that differentiate classic Hunner IC from other phenotypes of BPS/IC, in terms of age at first appearance of symptoms, endoscopic presentation, histologic features including mast cell expression, response to various treatments, and neurobiological findings [5, 7, 13–16]. That also includes notions on prevalence [7, 8].

A real turning point came in 2003 when Tomohiro Ueda organized a world meeting on IC in Kyoto. The amazing differences between centers, countries and continents were exposed. The first meeting of ESSIC took place in Copenhagen somewhat later that year and resulted in epochmaking publications [12, 17]. Initiatives by large organizations to establish guidelines followed and has had a great impact, including the AUA and EAU guidelines, among many other things including the notion that chronic pain might be a disease process in its own right [18–21].

29.3 Where Were We Off Base?

Pioneering attempts of ablation [1, 2] were depreciated or forgotten, much depending on the misconception that classic interstitial cystitis with Hunner lesions was an uncommon syndrome with unclear differences to the large population of patients suffering from bladder pain.

29.4 Where Do We Go from Here?

There are arguments for and against all available methods as to possible risks/advantages, like possible induction of bladder wall scarring, duration of remission after treatment and the prevalence of side effects. Comparable studies with long-range observation would be of interest. Recent interest in steroid injection of Hunner lesions can be traced to Schulte and Reynolds in 1956. Risk/benefit ratios of resection, fulguration, and steroid injection to treat Hunner disease remain to be determined [22, 23].

In the scientific community, treatment methods require high scoring in level of evidence to earn high grades of recommendation. Such grading depends on the outcome of RCTs. No such studies on local ablation in BPS/IC have as yet been accomplished but are eagerly awaited.

References

1. Kerr WJ. Interstitial cystitis: treatment by transurethral resection. J Urol. 1971;105(5):664–6.
2. Greenberg E, Barnes R, Stewart S, Furnish T. Transurethral resection of Hunner's ulcers. J Urol. 1974;111:764–6.
3. Fall M. Conservative management of chronic interstitial cystitis: transcutaneous electrical nerve stimulation and transurethral resection. J Urol. 1985;133:774–8.
4. Peeker R, Aldenborg F, Fall M. Complete transurethral resection of ulcers in classic interstitial cystitis. Int Urogynecol J. 2000;11:290–5.
5. Fall M, Johansson SL, Vahlne A. A clinicopathological and virological study of interstitial cystitis. J Urol. 1985;133(5):771–3.
6. Gillenwater JY, Wein AJ. Summary of the National Institute of Arthritis, Diabetes, Digestive and Kidney Diseases Workshop on Interstitial Cystitis, National Institutes of Health, Bethesda, Maryland, August 28-29, 1987. J Urol. 1988;140(1):203–6.
7. Peeker R, Fall M. Towards a precise definition of interstitial cystitis: further evidence of differences in classic and nonulcer disease. J Urol. 2002;167:2470–2.
8. Logadottir Y, Fall M, Kåbjörn-Gustafsson C, Peeker R. Clinical characteristics differ considerably between phenotypes of bladder pain syndrome/interstitial cystitis. Scand J Urol Nephrol. 2012;46(5):365–70.
9. Homma Y, Ueda T, Tomoe H, Lin A, Kuo H, Lee M, et al. Clinical guidelines for interstitial cystitis and hypersensitive bladder updated in 2015. Int J Urol. 2016;23(7):542–9. Epub 2016 May 24
10. Doiron R, Tolls V, Irvine-Bird K, Kelly K, Nickel J. Clinical phenotyping does not differentiate hunner lesion subtype of interstitial cystitis/bladder pain syndrome: a relook at the role of cystoscopy. J Urol. 2016;196(4):1136–40.
11. Chennamsetty A, Khourdaji I, Goike J, Killinger K, Girdler B, Peters K. Electrosurgical management of Hunner ulcers in a referral center's interstitial cystitis population. Urology. 2015;85(1):74–8. Epub 2014 Nov 5.
12. van de Merwe JP, Nordling J, Bouchelouche P, Bouchelouche K, Cervigni M, Daha LK, et al. Diagnostic criteria, classification, and nomenclature for painful bladder syndrome/interstitial cystitis: an ESSIC proposal. Eur Urol. 2008;53(1):60–7.
13. Fall M, Johansson SL, Aldenborg F. Chronic interstitial cystitis: a heterogeneous syndrome. J Urol. 1987;137:35–8.
14. Logadottir Y, Ehren I, Fall M, Wiklund NP, Peeker R. Intravesical nitric oxide production discriminates between classic and nonulcer interstitial cystitis. J Urol. 2004;171:1148–51.
15. Peeker R, Aldenborg F, Dahlström A, Johansson SL, Li J-Y, Fall M. Increased tyrosine hydroxylase immunoreactivity in bladder tissue from patients with classic and nonulcer interstitial cystitis. J Urol. 2000;163:112–5.
16. Peeker R, Fall M, Enerbäck L, Aldenborg F. Recruitment, distribution and phenotypes of mast cells in interstitial cystitis. J Urol. 2000;163:1009–15.
17. Nordling J, Anjum F, Bade J, Bouchelouche K, Bouchelouche P, Cervigni M, et al. Primary evaluation of patients suspected of having interstitial cystitis (IC). Eur Urol. 2004;45(5):662–9.
18. Engeler D, Baranowski A, Dinis-Oliveira P, Elneil S, Hughes J, Messelink E, et al. The 2013 EAU guidelines on chronic pelvic pain: is management of chronic pelvic pain a habit, a philosophy, or a science? 10 years of development. Eur Urol. 2013;64(3):431–9.
19. Fall M, Baranowski A, Elneil S, Engeler D, Hughes J, Messelink E, et al. EAU guidelines on chronic pelvic pain. Eur Urol. 2010;57(1):35–48.
20. Fall M, Baranowski AP, Fowler CJ, Lepinard V, Malone-Lee JG, Messelink EJ, et al. EAU guidelines on chronic pelvic pain. Eur Urol. 2004;46(6):681–9.
21. Hanno P, Burks D, Clemens J, Dmochowski R, Erickson D, Fitzgerald M, et al. AUA guideline for the diagnosis and treatment of interstitial cystitis/bladder pain syndrome. J Urol. 2011;185(6):2162–70.
22. Schulte TL, Reynolds LR. Transurethral intramural injection of hydrocotone hyaluronidase for interstitial cystitis (hunner's ulcers). J Urol. 1956;75:63–5.
23. Cox M, Klutke JJ, Klutke GC. Assessment of patient outcomes following submucosal injection of triamcinolone for treatment of Hunners ulcer subtype interstitial cystitis. Can J Urol. 2009;16:4536–40.

30 Treatment of Interstitial Cystitis with the Neodymium YAG Laser: A Swedish View

Magnus Fall

Shanberg et al. [1] were the first to use the YAG laser for BPS/IC. Based on observations in five patients they stated that treatment should be limited to those who are positively diagnosed and have failed more conservative forms of therapy. The results did not seem as beneficial for patients with intractable pain and signs of glomerulations only (at this time phenotyping was not part of the clinical routines). Rofeim et al. [2] presented a more recent prospective series of 24 patients with classic interstitial cystitis who had failed medical treatment, subjected to ablative therapy of their Hunner lesions by means of Nd:YAG laser. The power setting was 15 W. with a firing duration of between 1 and 3 s. All patients had symptom improvement within 2–3 days, including significantly decreased pain and urgency as well as substantial increase of voiding interval. There were no complications. Mean follow-up was 23 months, retreatment required in 11 patients. The re-treatment response was similar to the initial treatment.

Although the use of YAG laser has been more widespread than publications may suggest, the mode of ablation might be of secondary importance. Completeness of ablation may be the most important factor, irrespective of instruments used. Fulguration using various methods is today widely appreciated [3–6]. Simple coagulation is technically easier than resection and therefore preferred by most urologists, and is today standard treatment of patients with Hunner lesions (ESSIC type 3C).

Points of interest:

1. There are arguments for and against all available methods as to possible risks/advantages, like possible induction of bladder wall scarring, duration of remission after treatment and the prevalence of side effects. Comparable studies with long-range observation would be of interest.
2. In the scientific community, acceptance of methods depends much on the outcome of RCTs. No such studies on local ablation in BPS/IC have as yet been designed and accomplished but are eagerly awaited.

References

1. Shanberg A, Baghdassarian R, Tansey L. Treatment of interstitial cystitis with the neodymium-YAG laser. J Urol. 1985;134(5):885–8.
2. Rofeim O, Hom D, Freid R, Moldwin R. Use of the neodymium: YAG laser for interstitial cystitis: a prospective study. J Urol. 2001;166(1):134–6.
3. Payne R, O'Connor R, Kressin M, Guralnick M. Endoscopic ablation of Hunner's lesions in interstitial cystitis patients. Can Urol Assoc J. 2009;3(6):473–7.
4. Hillelsohn J, Rais-Bahrami S, Friedlander J, Okhunov Z, Kashan M, Rosen L, et al. Fulguration for Hunner ulcers: long-term clinical outcomes. J Urol. 2012;188(6):2238–41.

M. Fall
Department of Urology, Institute of Clinical Sciences, Sahlgrenska Academy at the University of Gothenburg, SE-41345 Göteborg, Sweden
e-mail: magnus.fall@urology.gu.se

P.M. Hanno et al. (eds.), *Bladder Pain Syndrome – An Evolution*,
https://doi.org/10.1007/978-3-319-61449-6_30

5. Chennamsetty A, Khourdaji I, Goike J, Killinger K, Girdler B, Peters K. Electrosurgical management of Hunner ulcers in a referral center's interstitial cystitis population. Urology. 2015;85(1):74–8. Epub 2014 Nov 5
6. Niimi A, Nomiya A, Yamada Y, Suzuki M, Fujimura T, Fukuhara H, et al. Hydrodistension with or without fulguration of Hunner lesions for interstitial cystitis: long-term outcomes and prognostic predictors. Neurourol Urodyn. 2016;35(8):965–9. Epub 2015 Jul 24.

Treatment of Interstitial Cystitis with the Neodymium YAG Laser: The Russian View

31

Andrew Zaitcev

31.1 What Did We Get Right?

Fulguration of Hunner lesions is specifically recommended for Hunner type IC with evidence level 3 or recommendation Grade B-C in clinical guidelines [1–4]. The introduction of the neodymium: yttrium aluminum-garnet laser (Nd:YAG) in 1985 by Shanberg and Malloy [5] offered the theoretical possibility of primary Hunner type IC or recurrent ulcer treatment. Authors have found it necessary to lower the wattage of energy used to prevent damage to structures adjacent to the bladder. Most patients (17 of 19) with Hunner lesion showed good results, but 12 reported recurrence of symptoms between 6 and 8 months' post-treatment. The outcome was worse in non-Hunner type of disease and did not exceed 65%. In two patients, small—bowel perforations occurred.

31.2 What Seminal Publications Changed Our Thinking?

A study by Chennamsetty et al. [6] reported that 89.6% of 76 Hunner type IC patients noted some degree of symptom improvement after fulguration and 98% of patients answered that they would undergo fulguration when symptoms recurred. Hillelsohn et al. [7] reported that 45.8% of 59 Hunner type IC patients required repeated fulguration with a mean time between fulgurations of 20.3 months. A recent study by Niimi et al. confirmed these observations with a larger sample size [8]. In our experience holmium: YAG laser seems preferable (with a power of 20 Watt, output energy of 3 J, wavelength of 2100 nm) for endovesical coagulation of Hunner's lesions. It is less dangerous and has the same efficacy [9]. Results showed a significant immediate reduction of pain and improvement of the quality of life of the patients. By using the usual parameters for tissue destruction (blanching without charring) the depth of thermal injury in the bladder was kept superficial. Note that when performing partial nephrectomies, a twofold reduction in the zone of coagulative necrosis was demonstrated compared to the use of the continuous wave Nd:YAG laser [10].

31.3 Where Were We Off Base?

The therapeutic failure rate is higher in non-Hunner type BPS. The mean time to therapeutic failure is shorter in patients with endometriosis, irritable bowel syndrome (IBS), pelvic congestion syndrome and other comorbid pain syndromes.

A. Zaitcev
Department of Urology, MSMSU, Moscow, Russian Federation
e-mail: zaitcevandrew@mail.ru

P.M. Hanno et al. (eds.), *Bladder Pain Syndrome – An Evolution*,
https://doi.org/10.1007/978-3-319-61449-6_31

31.4 Where Do We Go from Here?

Hunner lesion fulguration is an effective treatment for patients with Hunner type BPS/IC who are refractory to less invasive therapies. Approximately 50% of patients who undergo fulguration require a repeat procedure and most of these repeat procedures are done within 3 years of initial treatment. Further studies are required to obtain clear scientific evidence of the efficacy of this treatment modality. Meanwhile, new research should be performed in order to identify various clinical phenotypes and update classification systems based on the multimodal therapeutic approach and evaluation of patients.

References

1. van de Merwe JP, Nordling J, Bouchelouche P, et al. Diagnostic criteria, classification, and nomenclature for painful bladder syndrome/interstitial cystitis: an ESSIC proposal. Eur Urol. 2008;53:60–7.
2. Homma Y, Ueda T, Tomoe H, et al. Clinical guidelines for interstitial cystitis and hypersensitive bladder syndrome. Int J Urol. 2009;16:597–615.
3. Hanno PM, Burks DA, Clemens JQ, et al. AUA guideline for the diagnosis and treatment of interstitial cystitis/bladder pain syndrome. J Urol. 2011; 185:2162–70.
4. Cox A, Golda N, Nadeau G, Nickel JC, Carr L, Corcos J, Teichman J. CUA guideline: diagnosis and treatment of interstitial cystitis/bladder pain syndrome. Can Urol Assoc J. 2016;10(5–6):E136–55.
5. Shanberg AM, Malloy T. Treatment of interstitial cystitis with neodymium:YAG laser. Urology. 1987;29(4 Suppl):31–3.
6. Chennamsetty A, Khourdaji I, Goike J, et al. Electrosurgical management of Hunner ulcers in a referral center's interstitial cystitis population. Urology. 2015;85(1):74–8.
7. Hillelsohn JH, Rais-Bahrami S, Friedlander JI, et al. Fulguration for Hunner ulcers: long-term clinical outcomes. J Urol. 2012;188:2238–41.
8. Niimi A, Nomiya A, Yamada Y, Suzuki M, Fujimura T, Fukuhara H, et al. Hydrodistension with or without fulguration of Hunner lesions for interstitial cystitis: long-term outcomes and prognostic predictors. Neurourol Urodyn. 2016;35(8):965–9. Epub 2015 Jul 24.
9. Zaitcev A, Pushkar D, Diyakov V, Galchikov I. Use of Ho:YAG laser in the treatment of patients with recurrent and interstitial cystitis. Eur Urol Suppl. 2006;5(2):194.
10. Johnson DE, Cromeens DM, Price RE. Use of the holmium:YAG laser in urology. Lasers Surg Med. 1992;12(4):353–63.

32 Partial Denervation Procedures for Bladder Pain Syndrome

Rajesh Taneja

32.1 What Did We Get Right?

Partial denervation of bladder was used to treat severe urgency and urge incontinence in women and was first documented in the year 1959 [1]. Over the period of years, Ingleman and Sundeberg documented and advocated the efficacy of this procedure of partial denervation of the urinary bladder through the vaginal route [2, 3]. Cespedes and co workers published the results of the same procedure with minor modifications to treat urge incontinence in women [4, 5]. Rackley and Abdalmalak in their compilation of surgical management of overactive bladder have summarized the various possible denervation techniques of bladder for use in intractable cases [6].

32.2 Where Were We Off Base?

However, in none of the above-mentioned works, have authors mentioned the use of partial denervation for bladder pain syndrome. Over the period of last 30 years, the understanding of this disease entity has gone through a major evolution, with experts around the globe defining the Bladder Pain Syndrome (BPS) as a clearly demarcated entity different from overactive bladder. It has been clearly understood that the frequency and urgency in cases of BPS is primarily due to the pain or discomfort that the patient feels upon filling of bladder, and the fact that patient learns to get relief of pain/discomfort by will fully evacuating the bladder. This is a major deviation from overactive bladder in which the patient willfully is trying to prevent the emptying of bladder. Thus pain/discomfort perceived to be originating from the urinary bladder has now been recognized as pivotal to the definition of Bladder pain syndrome, erstwhile known as interstitial cystitis. Denervation procedures were aimed at reducing the frequency and urgency due to increased detrusor activity unrelated to pain.

R. Taneja
Urology, Apollo Hospital, New Delhi, India
e-mail: rajeshtanejadr@yahoo.com

32.3 What Seminal Publications Changed Our Thinking?

Towards the end of last century, it was recognized that the NIDDK criteria for interstitial cystitis were good for research purposes but were found to be restrictive when applied in clinical practice as was documented in the publication by Hanno et al. [7]. In another publication, the International Continence Society expressed the need for segregating painful condition of the bladder from overactive bladder (OAB) [8]. Publication of the proceedings during the international consultation

P.M. Hanno et al. (eds.), *Bladder Pain Syndrome – An Evolution*,
https://doi.org/10.1007/978-3-319-61449-6_32

on Interstitial cystitis held in Kyoto, Japan attempted to define the entity of bladder pain as important criteria for diagnosis of Interstitial cystitis [9]. The European society for study of interstitial cystitis clearly defined pain or bladder discomfort perceived to be originating from urinary bladder as the prerequisite for the diagnosis of Bladder Pain Syndrome [10]. These publications indicated that the condition of Bladder pain syndrome was not actually a problem of storage as perceived in OAB, but had pain as the primary reason for urinary frequency.

32.4 Where Do We Go from Here?

None of the major scientific associations issuing guidelines for treatment of BPS include denervation procedures as an option for treating BPS [11–13].

References

1. Ingleman-Sundberg A. Partial denervation of bladder. A new method for the treatment of urge incontinence and similar conditions in women. Acta Obstet Gynecol Scand. 1959;38:487–502.
2. Ingleman-Sundberg A. Urge incontinence in women. Acta Obstet Gynecol Scand. 1975;54:153–6.
3. Obrink A, Bunne G, Ingleman-Sundberg A. Urethral pressure in urge incontinence and after hypogastric blockade. Urol Int. 1978;33:107–10.
4. Cespedes RD, Cross CA, McGuire EJ. Modified Ingelman-Sundberg bladder denervation procedure for intractable urge incontinence. J Urol. 1996;156:1744–7.
5. Westney OL, Lee JT, McGuire EJ, Palmer JL, Cespedes RD, Amundsen CL. Long-term results of Ingelman-Sundberg denervation procedure for urge incontinence refractory to medical therapy. J Urol. 2002;168:1044–7.
6. Rackley RR, Abdelmalak J. Surgical management of the overactive bladder: evacuation disorders. In: Davila GW, Ghoniem GM, Nasseri Y, editors. Pelvic floor dysfunction: a multidisciplinary approach; 2008.
7. Hanno PM, Landis JR, Matthews-Cook Y, Kusek J, Nyberg L Jr. The diagnosis of interstitial cystitis revisited: lessons learned from the National Institutes of Health interstitial cystitis database study. J Urol. 1999;161(2):553–7.
8. Abrams P, Artibani W, Cardozo L, Dmochowski R, van Kerrebroeck P, Sand P. Reviewing the ICS 2002 terminology report: the ongoing debate. International Continence Society. Neurourol Urodyn. 2009;28(4):287.
9. Ueda T, Sant GR, Hanno PM, Yoshimura N. Interstitial cystitis and frequency—urgency syndrome (OAB syndrome). Int J Urol. 2003;10(Suppl):S39–48. Review
10. van de Merwe JP, Nordling J, Bouchelouche P, Bouchelouche K, Cervigni M, Daha LK, Elneil S, Fall M, Hohlbrugger G, Irwin P, Mortensen S, van Ophoven A, Osborne JL, Peeker R, Richter B, Riedl C, Sairanen J, Tinzl M, Wyndaele JJ. Diagnostic criteria, classification, and nomenclature for painful bladder syndrome/interstitial cystitis: an ESSIC proposal. Eur Urol. 2008;53(1):60–7. Epub 2007 Sep 20.
11. Nordling J, Wyndaele JJ, van de Merwe JP, Bouchelouche P, Cervigni M, Fall M. Bladder pain syndrome: a guide for clinicians. Springer; 2012.
12. Hanno P, Lin A, Nordling J, et al. Bladder pain syndrome international consultation on incontinence. Neurourol Urodyn. 2010;29(1):191–8.
13. Hanno PM, Erickson D, Moldwin R, Faraday MM, American Urological Association. Diagnosis and treatment of interstitial cystitis/bladder pain syndrome: AUA guideline amendment. J Urol. 2015;193(5):1545–53. doi:10.1016/j.juro.2015.01.086. Review

Surgical Therapy of Bladder Pain Syndrome

33

Tomohiro Ueda, Jørgen Nordling, Ralph Peeker, and Magnus Fall

Endoscopic techniques have been used extensively, however with mixed results, but are generally accepted now, when more selectively applied, taking the importance of adequate phenotyping of BPS/IC into account. Neurosurgical procedures have a decreasing role. Major surgery has an important but limited role; the various procedures are extensive and in principle irreversible for a condition that otherwise implies a very modest risk of death or life-threatening complications. Many factors must be taken into account. Apart from the more immediate problems intra- and postoperatively, there are less obvious ones like metabolic consequences [1] and the late development of cancer after incorporation of bowel into the urinary tract [2]. Since 1990 the attitude has not changed but rather been strengthened: reconstructive procedures have been and are still to be regarded as last resorts, to be used very selectively when there is nothing else with reasonable efficacy to be offered.

The decision of which type of reconstruction to choose in BPS/IC might be difficult, especially since a somewhat greater selection of methods has been used during the last decades. The judgement to perform a big operation evolves over a longer period of time and should always be preceded by thorough and appropriate patient counselling, to communicate not only possible gains but even more the potential risks with the procedure, and to give the patient realistic expectations. Every patient scheduled for a complicated reconstruction must be thoroughly assessed. He/she must cope with the long-term consequences; continent urinary diversion and cystoplasty both require a patient with cognitive ability and a good manual dexterity to be able to perform intermittent catheterization if and when necessary. A fact to discuss is the high risk of reoperation for patients with a continent cutaneous stoma. A careful preoperative assessment of renal and bowel function is a necessity when calculating the amount of bowel needed for the reconstruction [3]. In contrast to the urothelium the bowel mucosa has a significant permeability to ammonium chloride, the resorption of which may bring about hyperchloremic metabolic acidosis. A patient with compromised kidney function can have difficulties in compensating for this and as a consequence, continent urinary diversion can only be offered to patients with a glomerular filtration rate in excess of 40 mL/min/1.73 m^2 body surface. Furthermore,

T. Ueda (✉)
Ueda Cinic, Kyoto, Japan
e-mail: tom328177@gmail.com

J. Nordling
Department of Urology, Herlev Hospital, Herlev, Denmark

R. Peeker • M. Fall
Department of Urology, Institute of Clinical Sciences, Sahlgrenska Academy at the University of Gothenburg, SE 41345 Göteborg, Sweden

P.M. Hanno et al. (eds.), *Bladder Pain Syndrome – An Evolution*,
https://doi.org/10.1007/978-3-319-61449-6_33

the isolation of an ileal segment may compromise bile acid reabsorption which in turn may result in diarrhea and even, particularly in patients with preoperatively compromised anal sphincter function, anal incontinence [1]. Uptake of folic acid/cobolamin may likewise be compromised.

Cystoplasty with supratrigonal cystectomy is standard with a long tradition (see e.g. Kay and Straffon) [4–6]. In Chap. 22 of the book from 1990 it is stated that the "treatment goal is to convert a high-pressure, non-compliant, small capacity bladder to a low-pressure, compliant, high capacity reservoir". When sticking to that goal you are essentially on the safe side. In fact, our hard-earned experience is that the patient who definitely benefits from a major operation, with incorporation of bowel into the urinary tract, is the patient with end-stage classic interstitial cystitis and severely reduced bladder capacity, at the stage when bladder wall inflammation has burned out [7]. Before that fact is realized and severe symptoms rather than critical clinical parameters determine indications for surgery, frustration for the patient and the doctor is unavoidable [8] even with more extensive surgery including continent and incontinent urinary diversion [9].

33.1 What Did We Get Right?

A reconstruction allowing urethral voiding, when feasible, is always to be preferred and urethral sparing (and mostly also trigonal sparing) techniques were and are first choice. Caecocystoplasty, followed by the functionally preferable ileocystoplasty and later, for very special circumstances, the orthotopic bladder, follow that principle, with diversion as a second line alternative.

33.2 What Seminal Publications Changed Our Thinking?

Several studies presented since 1990 agree that patients with a preoperatively large bladder capacity are unsuitable for cystoplasty [7, 9, 10] and require contemplation of other measures, while patients with a small, contracted bladder do well.

33.3 Where Were We Off Base?

Generally speaking, many previous reports on major reconstructive surgery have failed to recognize the decisive importance of phenotyping of BPS/IC, and small patient series combined with short follow-up have made conclusions doubtful.

One technique increasingly used after 1990 deserves special mention. The pioneer of continent diversion professor N. G. Kock, working in our institution, translated his principles into diversion of urine [11]. This is an elegant way to spare the patient an external appliance with all its drawbacks. All varieties of continent diversion rest on the Kock principle. A fact that was made evident by time. However, there is a high risk of reoperations in patients with a continent cutaneous stoma, and in this context an important notion is that a follow-up report found that although some 90% of the patients with a Kock pouch had a well-functioning diversion, patients with benign functional or inflammatory diseases were distinguished by clearly more reservoir problems than patients with spinal cord injury or malignant disease [12]. Because of these experiences, by us continent diversion in BPS/IC is rare today.

33.4 Where Do We Go from Here?

A restrictive and critical attitude is wise when contemplating major surgery in BPS/IC. In one category there is no reason to hesitate, though, and that is in end-stage classic IC with scar contracted bladder. In this situation we preferably use ileocystoplasty, provided there are no specific contraindications. In a frailer subject a Bricker conduit may be chosen.

Being aware of differing opinions about the role of major surgery, e.g. usefulness of diversion, cystectomy/no cystectomy etc. our contention is that the decisive factor for a successful outcome, like in any measure in BPS/IC, is critical evaluation of the detailed and accurate diagnostic assessment.

References

1. Olofsson G, Fjalling M, Kilander A, Ung K, Jonsson O. Bile acid malabsorption after continent urinary diversion with an ileal reservoir. J Urol. 1998;160(3 Pt 1): 724–7.
2. Ali-El-Dein B, El-Tabey N, Abdel-Latif M, Abdel-Rahim M, El-Bahnasawy M. Late uro-ileal cancer after incorporation of ileum into the urinary tract. J Urol. 2002;167(1):84–8.
3. Mills R, Studer U. Metabolic consequences of continent urinary diversion. J Urol. 1999;161(4):1057–66.
4. Kay R, Straffon R. Augmentation cystoplasty. Urol Clin North Am. 1986;13:295–305.
5. Giertz G. Interstitial cystitis: 13 patients treated operatively with intestinal bladder substitutes. Acta Chir Scand. 1966;13:436.
6. Dounis A, Gow JG. Bladder augmentation: a long-term review. Br J Urol. 1979;51:264–8.
7. Peeker R, Aldenborg F, Fall M. The treatment of interstitial cystitis with supratrigonal cystectomy and ileocystoplasty: difference in outcome between classic and nonulcer disease. J Urol. 1998;159(5):1479–82.
8. Fall M, Nilsson S. Volume augmentation cystoplasty and persistent urgency. Scand J Urol Nephrol. 1982;16:125–2.
9. Rössberger J, Fall M, Jonsson O, Peeker R. Long-term results of reconstructive surgery in patients with bladder pain syndrome/interstitial cystitis: subtyping is imperative. Urology. 2007;70(4):638–42.
10. Nielsen KK, Kromann-Andersen B, Steven K, Hald T. Failure of combined supratrigonal cystectomy and Mainz ileocecocystoplasty in intractable interstitial cystitis: is histology and mast cell count a reliable predictor for the outcome of surgery? J Urol. 1990;144(2 Pt 1):255–8.
11. Kock NG, Nilson AE, Nilson LO, Norlén LJ, Philipson BM. Urinary diversion via a continent ileal reservoir: clinical results in 12 patients. J Urol. 1982;128:469–75.
12. Jonsson O, Olofsson G, Lindholm E, Tornqvist H. Long-time experience with the Kock ileal reservoir for continent urinary diversion. Eur Urol. 2001;40(6):632–40.

The Birth of Conservative Management, Prescription Drug Applications, and Pelvic Floor Physical Therapy

34

Rebecca Rinko, Nima Shah, Melissa Dawson, and Kristene Whitmore

34.1 Where Were We Off Base?

Although there is still much to learn about interstitial cystitis/bladder pain syndrome (IC/BPS), the options for treating the symptoms of the disease have expanded significantly over the last 30 years. Many of the newly accepted choices for managing IC/BPS symptoms are conservative measures that have become the mainstay of treatment for many patients. Much of the focus for treatment has been on the bladder. Another key component in the management of IC/BPS is to treat the pelvic floor along with the bladder.

34.2 What Seminal Publications Changed Our Thinking?

Thanks to the work that has been done by Dr. Mary P. Fitzgerald, Dr. Robert Moldwin, Dr. Barabara Shorter, Dr. Kristene E. Whitmore, and their colleagues, we have a better understanding of the role that conservative treatments have in symptomatic relief of IC/BPS. Their research and publications changed the way in which we treat patients and are sited throughout this chapter [1–8].

34.2.1 Complementary and Alternative Medical Therapies

Interstitial cystitis is complex and therefore requires a multidisciplinary approach to treatment. Strong evidence for complementary and alternative medical therapies is limited, but they have been found to be beneficial for treating patients with IC/BPS and other chronic pelvic pain syndromes (CPPS).

34.2.2 Dietary Modification

Dietary modification is considered standard IC/BPS therapy and is included in the American Urological Association guidelines. This elimination diet includes an avoidance of certain food types considered to be bladder irritants, including citrus, coffee, artificial sweeteners, alcoholic beverages, arylalkylamine- containing foods and tomato-based products which often exacerbate IC symptoms [4, 7, 9, 10]. It is recommended for each patient to have a dedicated

R. Rinko, D.O. (✉) • N. Shah, M.D.
M. Dawson, D.O., M.S.
Division of Female Pelvic Medicine and Reconstructive Surgery, Department of Obstetrics and Gynecology, Drexel University College of Medicine, Philadelphia, PA, USA
e-mail: rebeccarinko@gmail.com

K. Whitmore, M.D.
Division of Female Pelvic Medicine and Reconstructive Surgery, Department of Obstetrics and Gynecology, Drexel University College of Medicine, Chair of Urology and Female Pelvic Medicine and Reconstructive surgery, Philadelphia, PA, USA

P.M. Hanno et al. (eds.), *Bladder Pain Syndrome – An Evolution*,
https://doi.org/10.1007/978-3-319-61449-6_34

hour of teaching and assessment for food/beverage consumption and adequate nutrition, and to emphasize steady water intake to dilute urine and reduce constipation [8, 11]. Evaluation of food, symptom and voiding diaries are important to identify triggers and compose an individualized and effective elimination diet [11].

34.2.3 Physical Therapy

IC/BPS is often accompanied by hypertonic, hyperspastic myofascial tissue. Physical therapy can help reduce irritative voiding symptoms by realigning the bony pelvis as well as stretching and strengthening the muscles of the pelvis. Manual therapy, myofascial massage, Thiele massage, and muscle-energy techniques help stretch and strengthening the pelvic floor [6, 8]. Myofascial Massage was shown to be more effective than global massage in treating pelvic pain [2, 3]. Thiele massage was also beneficial in treating chronic pelvic pain, and the technique is often performed by certified pelvic floor physical therapists [12, 13]. Dilator therapy and myofascial trigger point wands have also been used successfully in treating chronic pelvic pain [14].

34.2.4 Biofeedback

Bladder retraining and biofeedback are methods for patient initiated control of voiding symptoms, IC/BPS, and pelvic pain [1]. Patients learn to control pelvic floor muscles through visual feedback to achieve conscious control over contraction and relaxation of these muscles with a goal to break the cycle of the spasm [6]. Biofeedback has minimal risks, is safe and has shown to be effective in treating CPPS [15].

34.2.5 CBT/Psychotherapy

Patients with IC/BPS have considerable cognitive and psychosocial changes, and have difficulty coping and have altered pain sensory mechanisms [16]. Changes, including improved coping strategies, can predict positive treatment outcomes by reducing helplessness, increasing perceived control, and decreasing pain catastrophization [17]. Contextual cognitive behavioral therapy (CCBT) may be particularly effective for those with change-resistant behavior as found in multi-problem cases [18]. CCBT incorporates principles of exposure, acceptance, cognitive de-fusion, mindfulness and value-based methods. Primary goals of treatment are to increase patients' psychological flexibility for dealing with unwanted experiences and improve their engagement in activities that are important, ultimately decreasing the disability associated with chronic pain [18, 19].

34.2.6 OMT

Osteopathic manipulative therapy (OMT) includes techniques of muscle energy, balanced ligamentous tension, myofascial release, and counterstrain to help treat symptoms of IC/BPS and stabilization of pelvic support and posture. The philosophy of whole body and individualized therapy is maintained through OMT [20]. Women with IC/BPS responded better to treatment with myofascial physical therapy than to global therapeutic massage [3]. Osteopathy has also been show to help those with chronic pelvic pain syndromes in addition to IC/BPS [21].

34.2.7 Acupuncture

Acupuncture has been well-accepted therapy for modulation of bladder storage and emptying functions. There has been evidence of subjective and objective improvement following acupuncture therapy, especially in patients with refractory IC/BPS [22, 23]. Posterior tibial nerve stimulation (PTNS) has been found to show improvement in nighttime voiding, bladder volume, IC problem and symptom indices, and health status scales scores in a small group [24]. Success rates have been found to be 60–80% improvement in leakage episodes, nocturia, daytime frequency, voided volume and number of pads used [25, 26].

Further studies utilizing PTNS for IC/BPS are pending.

Multimodal therapy requires strong patient driven coping mechanisms as well as patience and determination. By actively participating in care, patients maintain a sense of control and can improve coping mechanisms [7]. In a study comparing IC patients and age-matched healthy controls there was greater mean daily stress, with a significant relationship between stress and urgency [27]. Guided imagery has also been found to improve urgency and pain scores in patients [28]. Exercise, stress relief, sleep hygiene, and yoga are alternative methods to reduce stress in the hopes of decreasing the severity of symptoms.

34.2.8 Over the Counter Medications

Several over the counter medications have been found useful in reducing IC/BPS symptoms. CystoProtek® is an oral supplement. The active ingredients include glucosamine sulfate, 280 mg; chondroitin sulfate, 300 mg; Sodium Hyaluronate, 20 mg; quercetin, 260 mg; rutin, 40 mg. Glucosamine sulfate, chondroitin sulfate and Sodium Hyaluronate are glycosaminoglycans (GAG) that may help to protect the bladder lining. Quercetin, an antioxidant, and rutin, with ant-inflmmatory properties, reduce bladder inflammation. CystoProtek® 4 capsules per day decreased pain scores significantly [29].

Prelief® is another oral supplement comprised of calcium glycerophosphate. Prelief takes the acidity out of common IC/BPS dietary triggers including coffee, tomato sauce, fruits and wine. This treatment is directed to those patients whose bladder is sensitive to these triggers [6]. In patients who took two tablets before each meal for a total of 4 weeks, pain and discomfort and urgency were significantly decreased and quality of life was either the same or improved [30].

Another over the counter supplement is, Quercetin. Quercetin is a flavonoid found in many plants. With antioxidant qualities it is felt that the supplement help reduce irritative symptoms of IC/BPS. Patients who took 500 mg of quercetin twice a day for 4 weeks discovered symptom improvement [31].

34.2.9 Pharmacologic Treatment (Off Label Use)

The pharmacologic treatment of IC/BPS can be complex. Uribel® is an oral treatment that contains methenamine used to treat bladder discomfort, pain and frequent urge to urinate. Methenamine is an active ingredient in Uribel® and several other medications indicated for the treatment of recurrent UTIs. This anti-infective mechanism has been shown to prevent recurrent UTIs in women and is used in several formulations such as Urogesic-Blue™ for the treatment of IC/BPS although no studies have proved its efficacy in decreasing symptoms in this population [32, 33]. Similar medications such as phenazopyridine also reduce the urinary symptoms of IC/BPS by acting as a local analgesic to the bladder [34].

Antidepressants are used in the treatment of IC/BPS, although amitriptyline is the only drug that has been studied in chronic urological pelvic pain [35]. Duloxitine is a serotonin-norepinephrine reuptake inhibitor approved for the treatments of major depressive disorder, fibromyalgia and chronic pain and is used for the treatment of female stress urinary incontinence exclusively in Europe. It has been used in the treatment of IC/BPS [36]. Tricyclic antidepressants, specifically nortriptyline has been shown in a small study to decrease pain in women diagnosed with chronic pelvic pain [37].

Montelukast is a leukotriene receptor antagonist that may decrease the inflammatory process and improve bladder pain and urinary urgency while used in collaboration with other oral medications [38]. Diazepam is a well known for its antispasmodic activity in the treatment of muscle hypertonus and may also be effective in the treatment of IC/BPS [39, 40].

The Interstitial Cystitis Association (ICA) conducted an internet-based survey on complementary and alternative medical (CAM) therapies. Of those who responded, only 55% had physicians who recommended these therapies.

Patients considered physical therapy, heat and cold, meditation and relaxation, acupuncture, stress reduction, exercise and sleep hygiene as helpful. In addition, those who were recently diagnosed showed more improvement with therapies than those with a longstanding diagnosis [5]. This only affirms the need for physicians to discuss CAM therapies and to create an individualized therapeutic plan that is unique for the specific IC/BPS patient.

34.3 Where Do We Go from Here?

We have come a long way in our knowledge and understanding of IC/BPS. IC/BPS patients present with varying levels of pain and with various triggers. We can better serve our patients now, than ever before, using conservative and alternative treatments as an important part of the overall care plan. There are still areas of conservative and CAM therapies that are not well studied. Randomized control trials are needed to improve our use of all of these modalities. Other areas of interest for IC/BPS patients are the effects of different types of acupuncture, Chinese medicines, yoga, Reiki, meditation, hypnosis, different massage techniques, and guided imagery on symptom relief and pain management.

References

1. Atchley MD, Shah NM, Whitmore KE. Complementary and alternative medical therapies for interstitial cystitis: an update from the United States. Transl Androl Urol. 2015;4(6):662–7.
2. Fitzgerald MP, et al. Randomized multicenter feasibility trial of myofascial physical therapy for the treatment of urological chronic pelvic pain syndromes. J Urol. 2013;189(1 Suppl):S75–85.
3. FitzGerald MP, et al. Randomized multicenter clinical trial of myofascial physical therapy in women with interstitial cystitis/painful bladder syndrome and pelvic floor tenderness. J Urol. 2012;187(6):2113–8.
4. Friedlander JI, Shorter B, Moldwin RM. Diet and its role in interstitial cystitis/bladder pain syndrome (IC/BPS) and comorbid conditions. BJU Int. 2012;109(11):1584–91.
5. O'Hare PG III, et al. Interstitial cystitis patients' use and rating of complementary and alternative medicine therapies. Int Urogynecol J. 2013;24(6):977–82.
6. Wehbe SA, Fariello JY, Whitmore K. Minimally invasive therapies for chronic pelvic pain syndrome. Curr Urol Rep. 2010;11(4):276–85.
7. Whitmore KE. Self-care regimens for patients with interstitial cystitis. Urol Clin North Am. 1994;21(1):121–30.
8. Whitmore KE. Complementary and alternative therapies as treatment approaches for interstitial cystitis. Rev Urol. 2002;4(Suppl 1):S28–35.
9. Hanno PM, et al. AUA guideline for the diagnosis and treatment of interstitial cystitis/bladder pain syndrome. J Urol. 2011;185(6):2162–70.
10. Gillespie L. Metabolic appraisal of the effects of dietary modification on hypersensitive bladder symptoms. Br J Urol. 1993;72(3):293–7.
11. Gordon B, et al. Nutritional considerations for patients with interstitial cystitis/bladder pain syndrome. J Acad Nutr Diet. 2015;115(9):1372–9.
12. Oyama IA, et al. Modified Thiele massage as therapeutic intervention for female patients with interstitial cystitis and high-tone pelvic floor dysfunction. Urology. 2004;64(5):862–5.
13. Montenegro ML, et al. Thiele massage as a therapeutic option for women with chronic pelvic pain caused by tenderness of pelvic floor muscles. J Eval Clin Pract. 2010;16(5):981–2.
14. Anderson RU, et al. Equal improvement in men and women in the treatment of urologic chronic pelvic pain syndrome using a multi-modal protocol with an internal myofascial trigger point wand. Appl Psychophysiol Biofeedback. 2016;41(2):215–24.
15. Ye ZQ, et al. Biofeedback therapy for chronic pelvic pain syndrome. Asian J Androl. 2003;5(2):155–8.
16. Nickel JC, et al. Psychosocial phenotyping in women with interstitial cystitis/painful bladder syndrome: a case control study. J Urol. 2010;183(1):167–72.
17. Spinhoven P, Linssen AC. Behavioral treatment of chronic low back pain. I. Relation of coping strategy use to outcome. Pain. 1991;45(1):29–34.
18. McCracken LM, Vowles KE, Eccleston C. Acceptance-based treatment for persons with complex, long standing chronic pain: a preliminary analysis of treatment outcome in comparison to a waiting phase. Behav Res Ther. 2005;43(10):1335–46.
19. McCracken LM, MacKichan F, Eccleston C. Contextual cognitive-behavioral therapy for severely disabled chronic pain sufferers: effectiveness and clinically significant change. Eur J Pain. 2007;11(3):314–22.
20. Tettambel MA. An osteopathic approach to treating women with chronic pelvic pain. J Am Osteopath Assoc. 2005;105(9 Suppl 4):S20–2.
21. Marx S, et al. Chronic prostatitis/chronic pelvic pain syndrome. Influence of osteopathic treatment - a randomized controlled study. Urologe A. 2009;48(11):1339–45.
22. Geirsson G, et al. Traditional acupuncture and electrical stimulation of the posterior tibial nerve. A trial

in chronic interstitial cystitis. Scand J Urol Nephrol. 1993;27(1):67–70.
23. Katayama Y, et al. Effectiveness of acupuncture and moxibustion therapy for the treatment of refractory interstitial cystitis. Hinyokika Kiyo. 2013;59(5):265–9.
24. Zhao J, et al. Posterior tibial nerve stimulation twice a week in patients with interstitial cystitis. Urology. 2008;71(6):1080–4.
25. Govier FE, et al. Percutaneous afferent neuromodulation for the refractory overactive bladder: results of a multicenter study. J Urol. 2001;165(4):1193–8.
26. van Balken MR, et al. Posterior tibial nerve stimulation as neuromodulative treatment of lower urinary tract dysfunction. J Urol. 2001;166(3):914–8.
27. Rothrock N, Lutgendorf SK, Kreder KJ. Coping strategies in patients with interstitial cystitis: relationships with quality of life and depression. J Urol. 2003;169(1):233–6.
28. Carrico DJ, Peters KM, Diokno AC. Guided imagery for women with interstitial cystitis: results of a prospective, randomized controlled pilot study. J Altern Complement Med. 2008;14(1):53–60.
29. Theoharides TC, et al. Treatment of refractory interstitial cystitis/painful bladder syndrome with CystoProtek—an oral multi-agent natural supplement. Can J Urol. 2008;15(6):4410–4.
30. Bologna RA, et al. The efficacy of calcium glycerophosphate in the prevention of food-related flares in interstitial cystitis. Urology. 2001;57(6 Suppl 1):119–20.
31. Katske F, et al. Treatment of interstitial cystitis with a quercetin supplement. Tech Urol. 2001;7(1):44–6.
32. Aydin A, et al. Recurrent urinary tract infections in women. Int Urogynecol J. 2015;26(6):795–804.
33. Lee BB, et al. Methenamine hippurate for preventing urinary tract infections. Cochrane Database Syst Rev. 2007;(4):CD003265.
34. Hill JR, et al. Patient perceived outcomes of treatments used for interstitial cystitis. Urology. 2008;71(1):62–6.
35. Papandreou C, et al. Antidepressant drugs for chronic urological pelvic pain: an evidence-based review. Adv Urol. 2009;2009:797031.
36. van de Merwe JP, et al. Diagnostic criteria, classification, and nomenclature for painful bladder syndrome/interstitial cystitis: an ESSIC proposal. Eur Urol. 2008;53(1):60–7.
37. Walker EA, et al. An open trial of nortriptyline in women with chronic pelvic pain. Int J Psychiatry Med. 1991;21(3):245–52.
38. Traut JL, et al. Montelukast for symptom control of interstitial cystitis. Ann Pharmacother. 2011;45(9):e49.
39. Capra P, et al. Innovative approach for interstitial cystitis: vaginal pessaries loaded diazepam-a preliminary study. J Pharm (Cairo). 2013;2013:386546.
40. Rogalski MJ, et al. Retrospective chart review of vaginal diazepam suppository use in high-tone pelvic floor dysfunction. Int Urogynecol J. 2010;21(7):895–9.

Placing Interstitial Cystitis/Bladder Pain Syndrome on the Map: The Story of the Interstitial Cystitis Association

35

Vicki Ratner

Abstract

In 1984, interstitial cystitis (IC) was considered a rare psychosomatic disorder in post-menopausal women. In 2014, the Interstitial Cystitis Association of America (ICA) celebrated its 30th anniversary. We've come a long way since 1984 and great progress has been made. IC is now recognized as a condition. That afflicts both men and women of all ages, including children and teenagers. It is not a psychosomatic disorder. Though it was once thought to be an orphan Disease (defined as affecting less than 200,000 people), we now know that there are millions of women and men who suffer from IC/BPS (bladder pain syndrome). In looking back over the past 30 years, there were seven key reasons why the ICA Became so successful: an extremely dedicated ICA staff, Board of Directors and Volunteers, a very strong Medical Advisory Board and participation of many other Urologists from across the country and around the world; cooperation of the media; epidemiological studies; the ICA's Pilot Research Program; advocacy and our representation in Congress; and a strong working partnership with the National Institutes of Health (NIH). Great progress has been made, although we are still in the very early stages of understanding this disease, its causes, and finding treatments that are uniformly effective.

35.1 In the Beginning

In 1983, as a third year medical student, I came down with severe suprapubic pressure, urinary urgency, frequency and burning pain in my bladder. The pain felt like a lit match in my urethra. I was barely able to function, and found it almost impossible to concentrate. I assumed I had a UTI, but a complete work-up was negative and antibiotics failed to reduce the symptoms. In search of a diagnosis and relief from the severity of the symptoms, I sought help from one urologist after another—a total of 14. Many told me that the tests were negative and that there was nothing they could do for me. Others suggested that I was not cut out to be a doctor and that I should drop out of medical school, get

V. Ratner, M.D.
Founder and President Emeritus, Interstitial Cystitis Association of America, McLean, VA 22102, USA
e-mail: VRatner@aol.com

P.M. Hanno et al. (eds.), *Bladder Pain Syndrome – An Evolution*,
https://doi.org/10.1007/978-3-319-61449-6_35

married, and settle down into a more traditional lifestyle. I spent the last 2 years of medical school in intense, unremitting pain and isolation, imagining that I was the only one in the world with this disease.

Ultimately I made the diagnosis myself. While researching the problem in my medical school library (using Index Medicus at that time), I came across a footnote. It was almost 11 p.m., I was exhausted and ready to quit, the library was about to close. With little energy left after 2 days of searching, I pushed myself to stay, and to my amazement, that footnote led me to an article that described my case exactly. It was entitled "Early Interstitial Cystitis", published in 1978 by Ed Messing and Thomas Stamey, both from Stanford University Medical Center [1]. I was told by the chief resident of urology at my medical center at that time not to 'hang my hat' on just one article. It's a good thing I did.

Since my bladder looked normal during a routine cystoscopic procedure in the office, it took many months of convincing the urologist at my medical center to consider a cystoscopy under general anesthesia. The procedure was eventually done, according to the recommendations in the article I had found. The diagnosis was finally made based on numerous glomerulations seen on second distention of the bladder. (I realize that this does not necessarily meet today's criteria, but back in 1984 it did). For me, it was an enormous relief just to know that there was a name for what I was suffering from.

Prior to the mid-1980's, Interstitial Cystitis (IC) could still be found in the psychosomatic chapter on urologic conditions, described as a rare psychosomatic disorder which "may represent the end stage of a bladder that has been made irritable by emotional disturbances… a pathway for the discharge of unconscious hatred" [2]. In 1986, when the new edition of Campbell's Urology was published, IC was acknowledged as a real disease. The section on IC in the chapter on psychosomatic illness was removed, in fact the entire chapter was removed, prompted by a letter I had written in 1985 to the editors of Campbell's Urology.

35.2 Establishment of the ICA

In 1984, I was interviewed by WNBC news in New York City about IC. Among the many women who responded, all had a similar experience to mine, and a small group of us got together under my leadership, and we formed an organization called the Interstitial Cystitis Association of America. (ICA) I was doing my orthopedic surgery residency at that time, and taking charge of the ICA added an enormous amount of work to my already overwhelming schedule. We all suspected that there were many more patients out there suffering with the same symptoms, so we obtained official non-profit status in December, 1984, and founded *The Interstitial Cystitis Association of America.* Word spread to Philadelphia, and Phil Hanno, M.D. and his team of researchers at the University of Pennsylvania contacted me in the early spring of 1985 and we met to discuss IC, based on the responses we received from WNBC news and a recommendation from an IC patient that lived in Philadelphia.

Two weeks after we met, I was invited to be interviewed by ABC's *Good Morning America*, a very popular national morning show. Dr. Phil Hanno joined me. On the basis of a 5 min interview, the ICA received a response of over 10,000 letters during the first week alone. Over the ensuing 3 months, the ICA received over 100,000 letters. It was the largest phone response that "*Good Morning America*" had ever received, and they invited Dr. Hanno and me to be interviewed again 6 months later. This interview put the ICA "on the map."

35.3 The Patients

There were clearly thousands and thousands of women, and to a lesser degree men, who were suffering with nowhere to turn to for help. They had all gone through the same experience that I had: a negative work-up, told nothing was wrong or that the symptoms were all in their head. They had all seen numerous urologists. Their ages ranged from young to old, and many of the older patients had had symptoms for most of their adult lives. This was definitely not a post-menopausal disease. We now know that the average age of onset for this disease is 40 years old **(25% are under this age)**, and that it affects children and teenagers, although much less frequently.

In 1987, the following letter was syndicated nationwide:

> *Dear Ann Landers,*
> *"After three years of non-stop pain, 40–60 bathroom trips a day, little sleep, lots of tests, 12 doctors, hundreds of allergy shots, diets, antibiotics, and six unnecessary operations, I have finally been diagnosed as having interstitial cystitis, a 'rare' disease that doctors seldom look for and may turn out not be to so rare....*

35.4 The Doctors

Early on, despite most urologists still not believing their patients, a small group of extremely dedicated urologists and researchers began to work with the ICA in the capacity of the ICA's Medical Advisory Board. The earliest Board members were Drs. Phil Hanno (U. Penn), Alan Wein (Chairman, U. Penn), and Grannum Sant (Tuft's Medical Center). They gave us invaluable advice and opened many doors which would have otherwise been closed to us. With an ever increasing cadre of excellent researchers, many new theories on etiology and treatment are currently being evaluated.

35.5 What Did We Get Right?

Great strides have been made since 1984, when the Interstitial Cystitis Association of America (ICA), a non-profit advocacy group, was established. Since that time, there has been a substantial increase in awareness and understanding of Interstitial Cystitis/ Bladder Pain Syndrome (IC/BPS) and Chronic Prostatitis/Chronic Pelvic Pain (CP/CPPS) among general physicians, urologists, gynecologists, urogynecologists, as well as the public at large.

35.6 The Media

We could not afford to hire a public relations firm, so I personally wrote numerous letters to TV stations, newspapers and women's magazines in an effort to get media coverage about IC. At first, there were many rejections – "not for our audience," or "call back when you find a cure." It took a tremendous amount of perseverance to succeed in getting information about IC in print and on TV, and I did this entirely by myself.

I was ultimately extremely effective in "getting the word out" in both national and local television programs, national and local newspapers, and all the major national women's magazines. Once a story on IC was aired on the news, or an article appeared in print, patients were able to identify themselves (or their friends and relatives) and then contact the ICA. These people were then able to go to their doctors armed with information from the ICA and the media, for example, an article by Jane Brody from the *New York Times*. The doctors were then more likely to listen to the patients and believe them.

35.7 Had It Not Been for the ICA, Research Would Have Never Begun

35.7.1 On IC/BPS

The media, as mentioned previously, was critical in finding the IC/BPS patients nationwide. This led to the establishment of the ICA, whose goals were to educate both physicians, healthcare providers and patients about IC, provide support for patients, and raise funding for research. Our website, www.ichelp.org has a wealth of information, in addition to having a strong social media presence. We provide numerous brochures and fact sheets on a multitude of subjects, and respond to numerous letters and emails from around the world, as well as phone calls, which we usually receive from within the U.S. There are many state and local support groups for patients. As a result, patients learn so much from each other and feel much less isolated. In addition, the ICA produces a quarterly newsletter, and a monthly e-newsletter which updates physicians and patients on research and other important news.

The ICA has been instrumental in supporting IC/BPS research in several ways. Since the beginning, our own annual ICA Pilot Research Program has been very successful. However, these small grants, many of which have gone on to receive NIDDK funding, were hardly sufficient to ensure adequate funding for such a complex disease as IC/BPS. These ICA grants are only the first step. We needed the support of Congress, who controls the NIH (National Institutes of Health) budget.

35.7.2 Advocacy

Having found each other through the media, we learned that we were not alone, and knew much more about our condition then most doctors did. For example, IC patients were the first to figure out that there were other associated medical conditions, and the list is almost identical to the list that is used today [3].

Many patients from all types of backgrounds, whether they were housewives or teachers, nurses or secretaries, became activists and educators. We had a collective voice. This had a tremendous impact on NIH funding and policy for Interstitial Cystitis, much like the Breast Cancer Movement, the Aids Movement and many other patient organizations fighting for recognition of often lesser known diseases that they or a family member were afflicted with [4].

This collective voice had major political ramifications early on. Since its inception, the ICA has been extremely successful in testifying, lobbying and securing funding from Congress that has been dedicated specifically for IC/BPS research at the Division of Urology at NIDDK.

We were extremely fortunate that Senator Harry Reid (D) Nevada worked diligently with the ICA for over 25 years. During the early 1990s, several of the ICA staff and Board Members met with U.S. Senator Reid at his office in Nevada, and he took our cause very seriously. From that time on, he was always our champion. He made sure that funding was available for IC research, and that it went specifically towards projects that both the ICA and the Division of Urology had outlined. With the support not only of Senator Reid, but Dr. Lee Nyberg, Director of Urology at NIDDK, (now retired) and Dr. Chris Mullins, the current Director of Urology, we were able to get funding for IC specific research. As time progressed, Senator Reid became Majority Whip, and then Majority Leader of the Senate. It is most unfortunate that, due to a severe eye injury, Senator Harry Reid has had to retire. We will be forever indebted to him for his consistent and persistent work on our behalf.

35.7.3 International

Biannual conferences co-sponsored by the Division of Urology at NIDDK and the ICA over many years, as well as having an ICA booth at the annual AUA (American Urological Association) meetings, prompted many new researchers in urology in the United States and around the world to begin their own research on IC/BPS, its etiology, treatment and ultimately its cure. Patient groups similar to the ICA were established in Germany, Italy, Belgium, France and Japan, among others. Many of us work together. In 2009, The ICA as well as other patient organizations around the world, joined ESSIC (European Society for the Study of IC/BPS), a professional medical organization. What initially began as a European organization, has now expanded worldwide, although it retains its original name.

35.8 Where Were We Off Base?

It is too premature to conclude that IC/BPS be considered a systemic disease. Although it does have associated conditions, there are no biomarkers or other factors linking them all under a unifying condition. It has been noted that there are changes in the white matter and grey matter in the brain of IC/BPS patients. These changes are more likely to be a result of, not a factor in the etiology of IC/BPS. We have not been able to produce an animal model thus far. If we knew what caused IC/BPS, an animal model would make a great difference in testing treatments for the condition. Currently, the proposed animals are based on somatic or chemical models, however IC/BPS is a visceral pain condition, not a somatic one. And lastly, a mean symptom severity score of 4.3 (1–10) in the IC/BPS patient population is surely an underestimation.

35.9 Where Do We Go from Here?

Having reviewed many papers about the newer theories on the etiology of IC/BPS, the most promising idea comes from a fascinating paper on Familial Crohn's Disease, which was recently published in mbio—American Society of Microbiology in late 2016. The authors of this study found that in many cases, Familial Crohn's Disease is caused by a biofilm produced by three organisms: Candida Tropicalis, E. Coli, and S. Marcescens [5]. These organisms, including a fungus, work in concert to form a biofilm. A combination of organisms including a fungus, with the biofilm that they produce together on the lining of the bladder, could very well be the etiology of IC/BPS. In considering this mechanism, cultures would be negative, and the symptoms of IC/BPS would not respond to antibiotics. I hope that in the future, this area will be explored thoroughly.

Another etiology that appears to have been overlooked or dismissed is a theory that involves mast cells. It is worthwhile taking a second look. In the bladder, mast cells are in close proximity to neurons, as they are in all areas of the body. They all communicate with each other. Mast cells can both degranulate as well as transgranulate via the formation of filipodia (thin, finger-like projections) that attach directly to the neuronal membrane via endocytosis. The inflammatory mediators are released directly into the nerves of the bladder and could initiate and propagate the symptoms of IC/BPS via neurons in the bladder, which would then travel up the spinal cord to the CNS. Mast cells also degranulate directly into the bladder, and this could trigger symptoms as well. Some mast cells can even release inflammatory mediators without degranulation. Mast cells may be normal in number but could be hyper-responsive and degranulate more frequently than normal. This is another area that warrants investigation.

The MAPP studies (Multidisciplinary Approach to the Study of Pelvic Pain), which began in 2008 and should be concluded within 3 more years) will no doubt shed a great deal of light on IC/BPS. While it is important to acknowledge how far we have come, it is important to keep in mind how far we have to go, how much misery this condition is still causing, how many hundreds of thousands of lives it continues to ravage.

> *".....Part of the problem was that she was 65, and had probably had undiagnosed IC for almost 20 years....and was just diagnosed only 4 years ago.... I read the letter my mother left me. She was so sad to go, in fact did not want to go, but she could see no other way. She wasn't depressed or mentally ill at the time she made her decision..... Next to her bed was "The Final Exit", by Derek Humphry. While the doctors failed her, Mr. Humphrey gave my mother a way to end her pain easily, effectively, and quickly. It was a relief to learn that she did not suffer and it did not take long. But what a sad end to a vibrant woman's life! She was so very young for her age and it pains me to think of what IC took from her."*
> (Survived by 2 daughters and 2 grandchildren)

Acknowledgements A great deal of gratitude to Professor Gayle Greene, Scripps College, CA, for her excellent editing of this paper and to Gerry Buena, Independent Researcher, Stanford University.

Dedication This paper is dedicated to the many outstanding ICA staff, Board Members, volunteers, Medical Advisory Board Members, and to the many IC/BPS patients and urologists and other specialists worldwide, both past and present, who have worked with the ICA over many years. It is also dedicated to the millions of patients with IC/BPS who have endured an immeasurable amount of suffering, and to those who, unable to endure such suffering, found suicide as the only way out. And finally, this paper is also dedicated to Daniel Brookoff, M.D., (now deceased), who was one of the finest, most compassionate and extraordinary physicians I have ever known.

References

1. Messing E, Stamey T. Interstitial cystitis: early diagnosis, pathology and treatment. Urology. 1978;12:381.
2. Campbell's Urology edition: 1978–1985.
3. Alagiri et al. Interstitial cystitis: unexplained associations with other chronic disease and pain syndromes. Urology. 1997;49(supplement 5A):52–57.
4. Gayle G. Insomniac. University of California Press; 2008. p. 353–354.
5. Hoarau G, et al. Bacteriome and mycobiome interactions underscore dysbiosis in familial Crohn's disease. J Microbiology (mBio). 2016;7(5):1–11.
6. V.Ratner, Commentary: Mast Cell Activation Syndrome. Translational Andrology and Urology 2015; 4(5): 587–588.

Back to the Future: Looking Forward by Examining the Past

36

John W. Kusek and Chris Mullins

The plot for the classic movie, *Back to the Future*, begins with two of the main characters transported 30 years into the past. As the movie concludes they traverse 30 years into the future. We are taking a similar voyage in time with ***Bladder Pain Syndrome, Thirty Years Later***. Edited by long time leaders in the field, this unique volume takes the reader on a trip in a "time machine" through over 30 years of interstitial cystitis/bladder pain syndrome (IC/BPS) research and reveals based on what we know now "what we got right and where we missed the mark". Our contribution looks forward to examine the unmet needs of patients with IC/BPS for a number of important domains including etiology, diagnosis, prognosis, treatment, and prevention. We offer our comments on how these areas could be further investigated by adopting a more comprehensive approach [1] and applying new research technologies to this syndrome to propel us into the age of precision medicine [2]. An important goal in this journey is to identify the "right treatment for the right patient at the right time". This will require a substantial evolution of our knowledge. Given our current understanding and ongoing research efforts we believe that the time required for these advancements while significant, will be accelerated in the coming years, as new technologies and scientific strategies are applied to the study of this challenging syndrome. We anticipate this will be an exciting period of time as these research advances translate into significantly improved care of patients with IC/BPS and ultimately their prevention founded on identification of underlying risk and susceptibility factors.

36.1 Etiology

> *"Despite attempts of many workers to clarify matters, its (interstitial cystitis) etiology remains obscure"* [3].

IC/BPS remains an enigmatic syndrome. Although considerable effort has been expended over the past several decades to identify infectious and non-infectious causes for this syndrome none have emerged as leading candidates. Thus, the clinical diagnosis of IC/BPS remains mainly based on excluding known illnesses and conditions-the so-called "confusable diseases". This lack of precision in making a diagnosis undoubtedly leads to heterogeneity of patients and difficulty in matching the right patient with the right treatment. Thus, it is not surprising to observe use of multiple treatments in many patients and subsequent failed response to therapy. Importantly, the disappointing findings from many randomized clinical trials may

J.W. Kusek, Ph.D. (✉) • C. Mullins, Ph.D.
Division of Kidney, Urologic and Hematologic Diseases, National Institute of Diabetes and Digestive and Kidney Diseases, National Institutes of Health, Bethesda, MD, USA
e-mail: kusekj@extra.niddk.nih.gov; mullinsc@mail.nih.gov

P.M. Hanno et al. (eds.), *Bladder Pain Syndrome – An Evolution*,
https://doi.org/10.1007/978-3-319-61449-6_36

be the result of study designs involving such broad groups of patients with diverse causes of their symptoms.

We believe we are now embarking on a period of substantial discovery that will delineate pathophysiological factors underlying IC/BPS. Studies utilizing state-of-the-art technology to assess the urinary microbiome, [4], metabolome [5] and proteome [6] hold great promise to better understand biological factors that contribute to initiating disease and those that exacerbate established disease (e.g., precipitate symptom worsening). Non-biological factors, including psychosocial characteristics will likely add important insights [7]. Combining the findings from these various approaches, as well as genetic studies [8], will require application of sophisticated statistical techniques to complex data sets from large and well-designed studies of IC/BPS patients.

36.2 Diagnosis

"The diagnosis of BPS is thus made on the basis of exclusion of confusable diseases and confirmation by the recognition of the presence of the specific combination of symptoms and signs of BPS" [9].

As noted previously, IC/BPS remains primarily a diagnosis based on exclusion of other diseases and illnesses. The landmark 1988 publication of the National Institute of Diabetes and Digestive and Kidney Diseases (NIDDK) Consensus Criteria for the Diagnosis of Interstitial Cystitis ("the NIDDK Diagnostic Criteria") was an important first step to standardize the type of patients with IC enrolled in clinical research studies [10]. Subsequently it was recognized that applying these criteria was challenging. A report by Hanno and colleagues from the NIDDK-sponsored Interstitial Cystitis Database (ICDB) Study noted that upon applying these criteria more than 60% of patients traditionally classified by researchers as "definitely" or "likely" to have IC [11] would not have been included in this first ever major prospective study of IC. This observation and others resulted in a broadening of the NIDDK criteria for future research studies and ultimately to an expansion of the clinical spectrum of patients enrolled in clinical research studies of IC and the evolution of new terminology. As an example, the NIDDK Multidisciplinary Approach to the Study of Chronic Pelvic Pain (MAPP) Research Network describes IC/BPS patients (along with patients with chronic prostatitis/chronic pelvic pain syndrome [CP/CPPS]) under the new broader term Urologic Chronic Pelvic Pain Syndrome (UCPPS) [12, 13]. While not directly improving upon the diagnosis of IC/BPS this broadened designation has permitted a more comprehensive, less "bladder-centered" view of this syndrome. This idea that IC/BPS may involve systemic contributors has promoted the growing research trend toward more diverse, multi-disciplinary studies. At the forefront of this trend, the MAPP Research Network (http://www.mappnetwork.org/) is conducting highly integrated studies designed to identify underlying biological and non-biological factors contributing to IC/BPS development and progression and to aid in the classification of clinically relevant patient sub-groups. This involves a comprehensive examination of the urologic and non-urologic systems through epidemiological, neurological, and molecular approaches, as well as studies of animal models selected to mimic the human condition. The goal is to inform the next generation of clinical research studies, especially randomized clinical trials, and ultimately improve patient care through new insights.

36.3 Prognosis

"It's tough to make predictions, especially about the future", Yogi Berra

Despite the chronicity of IC/BPS surprisingly few studies have been conducted to determine factors that may predict future course. Such studies need to be relatively large, prospective in design, enroll participants with a broad range of clinical and demographic characteristics (age, symptom severity, time from diagnosis, etc.), collect extensive in-depth information (conduct "deep phenotyping" and apply new technology) and utilize state-of-the art statistical methods to fully characterize the features and clinical course of the participants. The first large-scale study to prospectively follow men and women with interstitial cystitis was the ICDB Study [14]. Although over 600 women and men with IC were enrolled in that study and followed for a median of 31 months, a high rate of lost to follow-up (31%) did not allow identification of factors predictive of symptom improvement or worsening. A decade later in 2008 a major new initiative on IC/BPS (and CP/CPPS), the MAPP Research Network [12, 13] was established. A major component of the now completed first phase of this multidisciplinary research program was a one-year longitudinal study of over 400 men and women with UCPPS. In the second phase, a larger (projected sample size to exceed 600) and longer (in some cases follow-up will be longer than 3 years) observational ("treated natural history") epidemiological study with extensive phenotyping is currently underway. Studies such as those conducted by the MAPP Research Network hold promise to determine whether characteristics measured at baseline and those assessed during follow-up can predict symptom progression and regression over time.

36.4 Treatment

> *"Although there are evidenced-based data supporting certain treatment approaches for (interstitial cystitis) patients in clinical studies, the unsolved question in clinical practice remains, 'Who is the ideal patient for a given treatment approach?'"* [15]

Clinical management of IC/BPS is undoubtedly in need of new insights. Nearly 20 years ago Rovner [16] and colleagues described the wide variety of treatments used for IC/BPS patients. Among the 581 women enrolled in the ICDB Study 183 different types of therapies were reported. A recent survey of urologists suggests that not much has changed in the intervening years. For example, at least 11 commonly used oral medications (range of frequency of use from 4 to 91%) were reported for treatment of IC/BPS, in addition to intravesical therapy and hydrodistension [17]. While guidelines for treatment are available in the United States [15], Canada, [18] and Europe [19] they are based primarily on low quality evidence, often from small and/or inadequately designed clinical trials. The disappointing results of many of these clinical trials are likely due, in large part, to inadequate methods of patient selection/sub-grouping resulting in heterogeneity of the treated group, absence of likely therapeutic targets due to lack of understanding of the underlying pathophysiology, and inadequate outcome measures (e.g., use of outcomes that combine both urinary and pain symptoms) [20], among other factors. Although there are investigational drugs for IC/BPS [21] the data necessary for evidence-based treatment recommendations will require a new generation of rigorously designed clinical trials to fully evaluate their efficacy.

36.5 Prevention

> *"An ounce of prevention is worth a pound of cure".*
> Benjamin Franklin

The ultimate goal of our efforts should be to prevent IC/BPS before symptoms manifest. To achieve primary and secondary prevention is a long-term proposition. However, tertiary prevention (e.g., reduction of pain and urinary symptoms) is within reach over the shorter term. Prevention of non-malignant urologic syndromes and diseases before these conditions become established and thus require treatment has received little attention. Noteworthy, the NIDDK Prevention of Lower Urinary Tract Symptoms (PLUS) Network has begun to lay the groundwork to prevent lower urinary tract symptoms and promote bladder health in women and girls [22]. It is anticipated that findings from the PLUS Network and other similar research will inform future efforts for secondary and possibly primary prevention of IC/BPS.

Conclusion

We are in the early stages of an exciting period of substantial progress in our clinical and mechanistic understanding of IC/BPS. Among many advances on the horizon, it is anticipated that ongoing research will yield new classifications of clinically meaningful patient sub-groups or phenotypes. Such phenotypes will need to be further evaluated for their ability to inform prognosis and for their response to targeted therapy. Once the clinical utility and underlying biology of these phenotypes are further established additional opportunities for addressing prevention are also possible. As we move toward the future using the lessons of the past, such endeavors will lead to clinical trials and prevention efforts based on a much stronger knowledge foundation and ultimately—and most importantly—improved clinical care for patients.

References

1. Bavendam TG, Norton JM, Kirkali Z, et al. Advancing a comprehensive approach to the study of lower urinary tract symptoms. J Urol. 2016;196:1342–9.
2. Collins FS, Varmus H. A new initiative on precision medicine. N Engl J Med. 2015;372:793–5.
3. Messing EM, Stamey TA. Interstitial cystitis. Early diagnosis, pathology and treatment. J Urol. 1978;12:381–92.
4. Nickel JC, Stephens A, Landis JR, et al. Assessment of the lower urinary tract microbiota during symptom flare in women with urologic chronic pelvic pain syndrome: a MAPP Network study. J Urol. 2016;195:356–62.
5. Parker KS, Crowley JR, Stephens-Shields AJ, et al. Urinary metabolomics identifies a molecular correlate of interstitial cystitis/bladder pain syndrome in a multidisciplinary approach to the study of chronic pelvic pain (MAPP) research Network cohort. EBioMedicine. 2016;7:167–74.
6. Chen Z, Kim J. Urinary proteomics and metabolomics studies to monitor bladder health and urological diseases. BMC Urol. 2016; doi:10.1186/s12894-016-0129-7.
7. Kanter G, Volpe KA, Dunivan GC, et al. Important role of physicians in addressing psychological aspects of interstitial cystitis/bladder pain syndrome (IC/BPS): a qualitative analysis. Int Urogynecol J. 2016; doi:10.1007/s00192-016-3109-2.
8. Manzoni C, Kia DA, Vandrovcova J, et al. Genome, transcriptome and proteome: the rise of omics data and their integration in biomedical sciences. Brief Bioinform. 2016; doi:10.1093/bib/bbw114.
9. Van de Merwe JP, Nordling J, Bouchelouche P, et al. Diagnostic criteria, classification, and nomenclature for painful bladder syndrome/interstitial cystitis: an ESSIC proposal. Eur Urol. 2008;53:60–7.
10. Gillenwater JY, Wein AJ. Summary of the National Institute of Arthritis, Diabetes, Digestive and Kidney Diseases workshop on interstitial cystitis. National Institutes of Health, Bethesda, Maryland, August 28-29, 1987. J Urol. 1988;140:203–6.
11. Hanno PM, Landis JR, Matthews-Cook Y, et al. The diagnosis of interstitial cystitis revisited: lesson learned from the National Institutes of Health interstitial cystitis database study. J Urol. 1999;161:553–7.
12. Clemens JQ, Mullins C, Kusek JW, et al. The MAPP Research Network: a novel study of urologic chronic pelvic pain syndromes. BMC Urol. 2016. http://www.biomedcentral.com/1471-2490/14/57.
13. Landis JR, Williams DA, Lucia MS, et al. The MAPP Research Network: design, patient characterization and operations. BMC Urol. 2016. http://www.biomedcentral.com/1471-2490/14/58.
14. Propert KJ, Schaeffer AJ, Bresinger CM, et al. A prospective study of interstitial cystitis: results of longitudinal followup of the interstitial cystitis data base cohort. The Interstitial Cystitis Data Base Study Group. J Urol. 2000;163:1434–9.
15. Hanno PM, Burks DA, Clemens JQ et al. American Urological Association (AUA) Guideline. Diagnosis and treatment of interstitial cystitis/bladder pain syndrome. 2014; 45 pages.
16. Rovner E, Propert KJ, Brensinger C, et al. Treatments used in women with interstitial cystitis: the Interstitial Cystitis Data Base (ICDB) Study experience. Urology. 2000;56:940–5.
17. Kivlin D, Lim C, Ross C, et al. The diagnosis and treatment patterns of urologists in the United States for interstitial cystitis/painful bladder syndrome. Urol Pract. 2016;3:309–14.
18. Cox A, Golda N, Nadeau G, et al. CUA guideline: diagnosis and treatment of interstitial cystitis/bladder pain syndrome. Can Urol Assoc J. 2016;10:E136–55.
19. Fall M, Baranowski AP, Elneil S, et al. EAU guidelines on chronic pelvic pain. Eur Urol. 2010;57:35–48.
20. Griffith JW, Stephens-Shields AJ, Hou X, et al. Pain and urinary symptoms should not be combined into a single score: psychometric findings from the MAPP Research Network. J Urol. 2016;195:949–54.
21. Chuang Y-C, Chermansky C, Kashyap M, et al. Investigational drugs for bladder pain syndrome (BPS)/interstitial cystitis (IC). Expert Opin Investig Drugs. 2016;25:521–9.
22. Bavendam TG, Star RA, Rodgers GP. Research to improve urological health for women and girls: focus on prevention. J Women's Health. 2016;25:1081–2.

37 Afterword

Philip Hanno and Alan Wein

It's been over 40 years since we first began doing basic infection research in the urology laboratory of the Harrison Department of Surgical Research at the University of Pennsylvania, following the work of Grant Mulholland, Lowell Parsons, Robert Levin, and Stan Shrom. We studied bladder antibacterial defense mechanisms, concentrating on the bladder surface lining. This evolved into our focus on possible bladder lining abnormalities in interstitial cystitis. At that time, there was only one FDA-approved therapy for this condition, intravesical application of dimethyl sulfoxide. It took 20 years for FDA approval of the next medication, the oral drug pentosan polysulfate. Neither medication has lived up to our hopes for a reliable treatment for this disease. None of the many therapies we commonly use have cleared the admittedly low bar of safety and placebo comparison necessary for FDA approval for this indication.

So, what is the problem? Is it the difficulty of discovering a treatment, or is it the description of the problem itself? Disease is defined as "a disorder of structure or function in a human, animal, or plant, especially one that produces specific signs or symptoms or that affects a specific location and is not simply a direct result of physical injury." A syndrome is "a group of symptoms that consistently occur together or a condition characterized by a set of associated symptoms." Hunner lesion could be a disease while bladder pain syndrome is just what its name implies. Syndromes and diseases are artificial descriptions of a condition designed to make it easier to help a patient who is sick. They can be considered as man-made constructs, and if the construct is not accurate, cure can be difficult to find. Does our lack of success reflect failure to find a cure or rather failure to appropriately define the illness? Time will tell.

Over the last 40 years there has been surprisingly little substantive advance in the diagnosis or patient care for most persons suffering with bladder pain syndrome. There has been a tremendous amount of money spent to advance the field. Much descriptive literature and data mining has been published, accounting for a major portion of the funds spent. On the positive side, recognition of the syndrome is much greater among providers and patients. There have been attempts to re-conceptualize "interstitial cystitis," most recently as urologic chronic pelvic pain syndrome. In some ways, this has only served to confuse the subject and make interpretation of the data more difficult. The search for a specific and sensitive biologic marker continues.

P. Hanno
Stanford University School of Medicine,
Stanford, CA, USA
e-mail: pmhanno@stanford.edu

A. Wein (✉)
University of Pennsylvania School of Medicine,
Philadelphia, PA, USA
e-mail: Alan.wein@uphs.upenn.edu

P.M. Hanno et al. (eds.), *Bladder Pain Syndrome – An Evolution*,
https://doi.org/10.1007/978-3-319-61449-6_37

We still hope for a breakthrough, and the avenue may be through phenotyping studies that show the value in isolating various patient clusters that may be diagnosed with more specificity and hopefully shown to respond better to specific therapeutic interventions. There is still a long way to go. For now, treatment remains an art, and a well-educated patient and specialty provider can work together to successfully improve quality of life.

This publication, 30 years after the initial monograph, reflects the efforts of the many patients, researchers, and clinicians trying to unravel the mystery and help those who are ill with bladder pain syndrome. We would like to thank our fellow editors and the members of the International Society for the Study of Bladder Pain Syndrome who made this volume possible and who devote much of their time to helping patients with chronic bladder pain.

Addendum 1: International Consultation

Reprinted with Permission of the International Consultation on Urological Diseases and the International Continence Society

Hanno PM, Cervigni M, Dinis P, Lin A, Nickel JC, Nordling J, van Ophoven A, Ueda T. Bladder pain syndrome. In: Abrams P, Cardozo L, Wagg A, Wein A, editors. Incontinence. 6th ed. London: ICS and ICUD; 2017. Chapter 19, 2203-2302. ISBN: 978-0-9569607-3-3

1.1.1 Definition

Bladder Pain Syndrome (in the absence of a universally agreed definition, the International Society for the Study of Bladder Pain Syndrome—ESSIC definition is given [1].

ESSIC: *Chronic pelvic pain, pressure or discomfort of greater than 6 months duration perceived to be related to the urinary bladder accompanied by at least one other urinary symptom like persistent urge to void or urinary frequency. Confusable diseases as the cause of the symptoms must be excluded.*

There is no published data as to what duration of symptomatology indicates that early spontaneous resolution of symptoms is unlikely. While ESSIC arbitrarily uses a 6 month duration, the American Urological Association Guideline suggests 6 weeks is long enough to initiate diagnosis and treatment of BPS [2]. Without further data, the Consultation cannot make a recommendation and believes that it is up to the discretion of the physician and patient as to the proper interval between symptom onset and evaluation and diagnosis of a chronic condition.

1.1.2 Bladder Pain Syndrome (BPS)

1.1.2.1 Nomenclature

The scientific committee of the International Consultation voted to use the term "bladder pain syndrome" for the disorder that has been commonly referred to as interstitial cystitis (IC). The term painful bladder syndrome was dropped from the lexicon. The term IC implies an inflammation within the wall of the urinary bladder, involving gaps or spaces in the bladder tissue. This does not accurately describe the majority of patients with this syndrome. Painful Bladder Syndrome, as defined by the International Continence Society, is too restrictive for the clinical syndrome.

Properly defined, the term Bladder Pain Syndrome appears to fit in well with the taxonomy of the International Association for the Study of Pain (IASP) (see below), and focuses on the actual symptom complex rather than what appears to be long-held misconception of the underlying pathology.

1.1.3 Bladder Pain Syndrome (XXIII-2) (per IASP)

Bladder pain syndrome is the occurrence of persistent or recurrent pain perceived in the urinary bladder region, accompanied by at least one other symptom, such as pain worsening with bladder filling and day-time and/or night-time urinary frequency. There is no proven infection or other obvious local pathology. Bladder pain syndrome is often associated with negative cognitive, behavioral, sexual, or emotional consequences as

P.M. Hanno et al. (eds.), *Bladder Pain Syndrome – An Evolution*,
https://doi.org/10.1007/978-3-319-61449-6

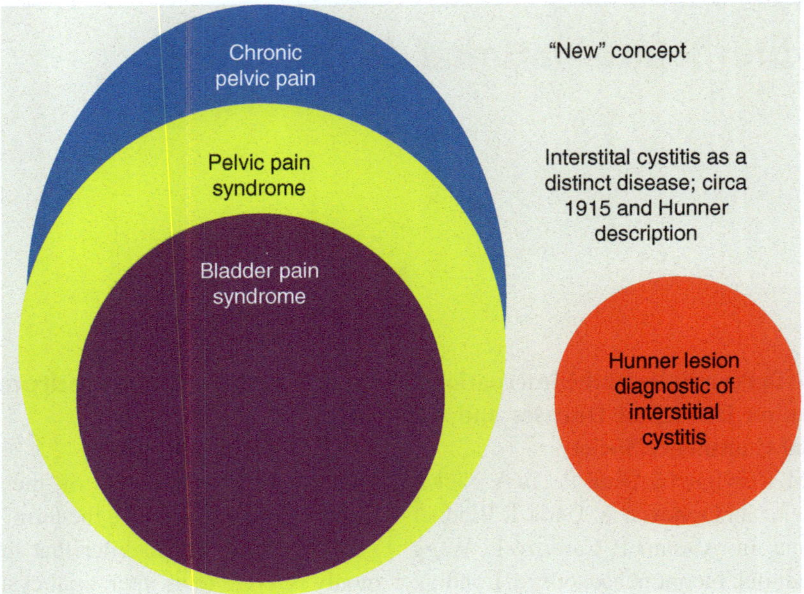

Fig. A1 Conceptualization of bladder pain syndrome vis a vis interstitial cystitis

well as with symptoms suggestive of lower urinary tract and sexual dysfunction.

The Consultation believes that based on the pathology and endoscopic findings characteristic of the Hunner lesion, the epidemiologic pattern that distinguishes it from bladder pain syndrome, the clinical response to local treatment of the lesion by resection, fulguration, or steroid injection, the response to cyclosporine, and the absence of reports in the literature that non-Hunner patients go on to develop Hunner lesions (i.e., the finding of Hunner lesion does not represent a continuum in the natural history of bladder pain syndrome), **the presence of a Hunner lesion should be considered a distinct disease**. It therefore should drop out of the bladder pain syndrome construct, much like we do not consider other painful conditions like radiation cystitis, ketamine cystitis, or urinary tract infection a part of bladder pain syndrome.

The Consultation concludes that it would be reasonable to designate the Hunner lesion in symptomatic patients with the term "interstitial cystitis", thus indicating a true interstitial inflammation. It would be defined much as Hunner defined it 100 years ago, and harmonize to a great extent the Asian, European, and North American concepts of interstitial cystitis. The Consultation will continue to refer to the symptom complex as "bladder pain syndrome". Hunner lesion will be considered a distinct phenotype, but in the future may be classified as a separate disorder entirely, albeit with local symptoms that are difficult to differentiate from bladder pain syndrome in the absence of endoscopy. In other words, we may be coming full circle in the historical perspective (Fig. A1).

1.1.3.1 History/Initial Assessment

Males or females whose symptoms meet the requirements of the definition of bladder pain syndrome should be evaluated. The presence of commonly associated disorders including irritable bowel syndrome, chronic fatigue syndrome, and fibromyalgia in the presence of the cardinal symptoms of bladder pain syndrome also suggests the diagnosis. Abnormal gynecologic findings in women and well-characterized confusable diseases that may explain the symptoms must be ruled out.

The initial assessment consists of a frequency/volume chart, focused physical examination, urinalysis, and urine culture. In the absence of confusable disorders (uncomplicated disease), a diagnosis can be made and treatment instituted. Urine cytology, cystoscopy, and urodynamic evaluation are recommended if clinically indicated and/or the diagnosis is in doubt (complicated disease). Patients with urinary infection should be treated and reassessed. Those with recurrent urinary infection, abnormal urinary cytology, and microscopic or gross hematuria are evaluated with appropriate imaging and endoscopic procedures, and only if findings are unable to explain the symptoms, are they diagnosed with BPS. **Grade of recommendation: C**

1.1.3.2 Initial Treatment

- Patient education,
- dietary manipulation,
- nonprescription analgesics,
- stress reduction,
- pelvic floor relaxation techniques comprise the initial treatment of BPS. In the patient with findings suggesting pelvic floor dysfunction, pelvic floor physical therapy with myofascial trigger point release and intravaginal Thiele massage is often an effective therapeutic intervention. **The treatment of pain** needs to be addressed directly, and in some instances referral to an anesthesia/pain center can be an appropriate early step in conjunction with ongoing treatment of the syndrome.

When conservative therapy fails or symptoms are severe and conservative management is unlikely to succeed,

- oral medication or
- intravesical treatment can be prescribed. It is recommended to initiate a single form of therapy and observe results, adding other modalities or substituting other modalities as indicated by degree of response or lack of response to treatment. **Grade of recommendation: C**

1.1.3.3 Secondary Assessment

If initial oral or intravesical therapy fails, *or before beginning such therapy based on clinician judgment,* it is reasonable to consider **further evaluation** which can include Urodynamics, pelvic imaging, and cystoscopy with bladder distention and possible bladder biopsy under anesthesia.

- Findings of bladder overactivity suggest a trial of antimuscarinic therapy.
- The presence of a Hunner lesion suggests therapy with transurethral resection, fulguration of the lesion, or direct steroid injection into the lesion.
- Distention itself can have therapeutic benefit in 30–50% of patients, though benefits rarely persist for longer than a few months. **Grade of recommendation: C**

1.1.3.4 Refractory BPS

Those patients with persistent, unacceptable symptoms despite oral and/or intravesical therapy are candidates for more aggressive modalities. Many of these/ are best administered within the context of a clinical trial if possible. These may include

- neuromodulation,
- intradetrusor botulinum toxin,
- oral cyclosporine A, or
- clinical trials of newly described pharmacologic management techniques. At this point, most patients will benefit from the expertise of an
- anesthesia pain clinic.

The last step in treatment is usually some type of surgical intervention aimed at increasing the functional capacity of the bladder or diverting the urinary stream.

- Urinary diversion with or without cystectomy has been used as a last resort with good results in selected patients. Cystectomy and urethrectomy do not appear to add any additional efficacy to diversion alone [3–5].
- Augmentation or substitution cystoplasty seems less effective and more prone to recurrence of chronic pain in small reported series. **Grade of recommendation: C**
- Pain management is a primary consideration at every step of algorithm
- Patient enrollment in appropriate research trial is reasonable option at any point
- Evidence supporting neurostimulation, cyclosporine A, and botulinum toxin for BPS indication remains limited. These interventions are appropriate only for practitioners with experience treating BPS and willing to provide long-term care post-intervention.

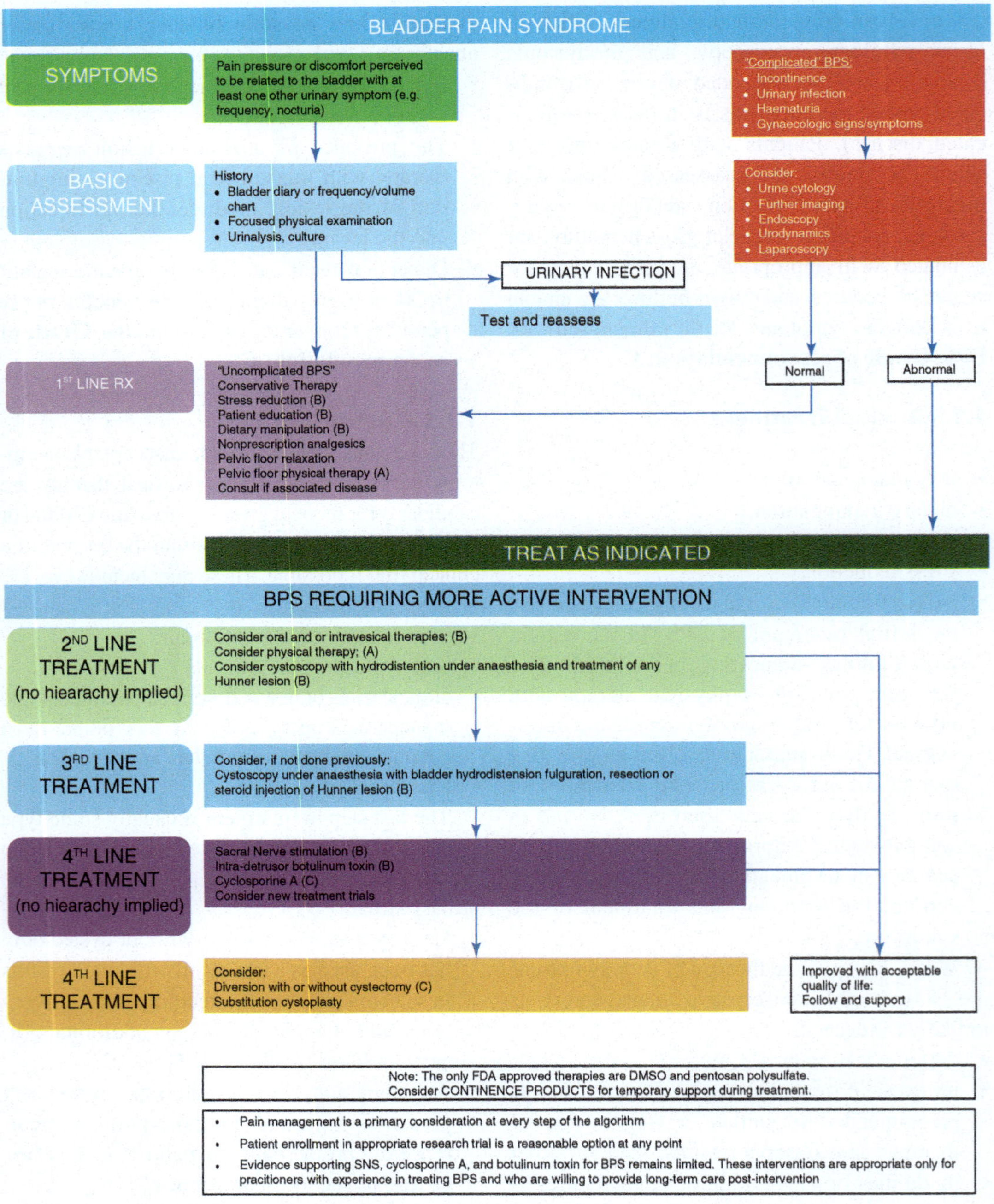

Algorithm for diagnosis and treatment: 2016 International consultation on incontinence

Bibliography

1. van de Merwe JP, Nordling J, Bouchelouche P, Bouchelouche K, Cervigni M, Daha LK, et al. Diagnostic criteria, classification, and nomenclature for painful bladder syndrome/interstitial cystitis: an ESSIC proposal. Eur Urol. 2008;53(1):60–7.
2. Hanno PM, Erickson D, Moldwin R, Faraday MM. Diagnosis and treatment of interstitial cystitis/bladder pain syndrome: AUA guideline amendment. J Urol. 2015;193(5):1545–53.
3. Andersen AV, Granlund P, Schultz A, Talseth T, Hedlund H, Frich L. Long-term experience with surgical treatment of selected patients with bladder pain syndrome/interstitial cystitis. Scand J Urol Nephrol. 2012;46(4):284–9.
4. Norus T, Fode M, Nordling J. Ileal conduit without cystectomy may be an appropriate option in the treatment of intractable bladder pain syndrome/interstitial cystitis. Scand J Urol. 2014;48(2):210–5.
5. Yang TX, Luo DY, Li H, Wang KJ, Shen H. Is urethrectomy necessary during cystectomy in patients with interstitial cystitis/bladder pain syndrome? Urology. 2016;97:73–9.

Addendum 2: AUA Guideline

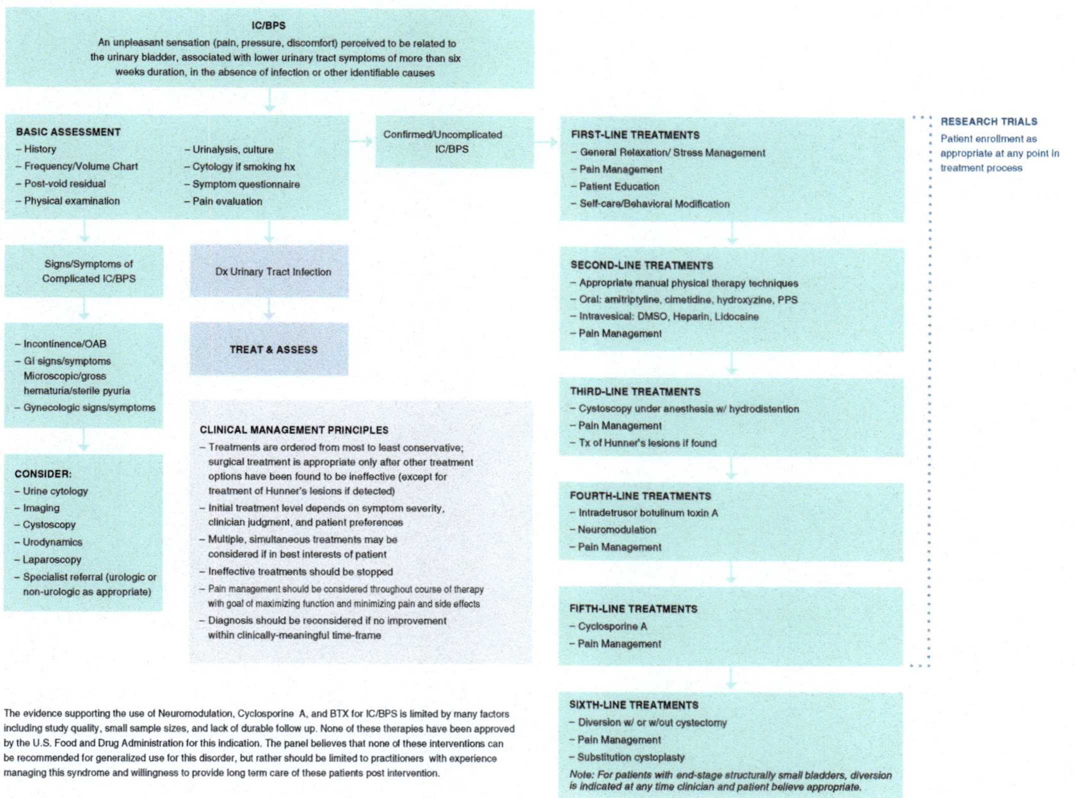

Guideline of the American Urological Association. Hanno PM, Erickson D, Moldwin R, Faraday MM: Diagnosis and treatment of interstitial cystitis/bladder pain syndrome: AUA guideline amendment. J. Urol. 193:1545-53, 2015

P.M. Hanno et al. (eds.), *Bladder Pain Syndrome – An Evolution*,
https://doi.org/10.1007/978-3-319-61449-6

Addendum 3: Asian Algorithm

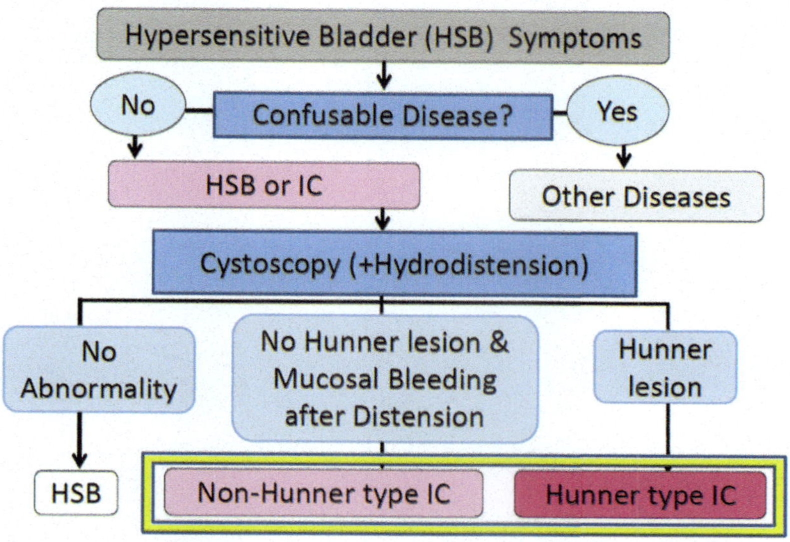

Asian conception of bladder pain syndrome from Homma. Homma Y, Ueda T, Tomoe H, Lin A, Kuo HC, Lee MH, Oh SJ, Kim JC, and Lee KS: Clinical guidelines for interstitial cystitis and hypersensitive bladder updated in 2015. International Journal of Urology. 23:542-549, 2016

P.M. Hanno et al. (eds.), *Bladder Pain Syndrome – An Evolution*,
https://doi.org/10.1007/978-3-319-61449-6

The manufacturer's authorised representative in the EU is Springer Nature Customer Service Centre GmbH, Europaplatz 3, 69115 Heidelberg, Germany. If you have any concerns regarding our products, please contact ProductSafety@springernature.com

Printed and bound by CPI Group (UK) Ltd, Croydon, CR0 4YY

22/09/2026

02220957-0014